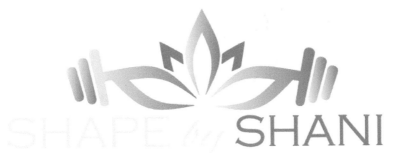

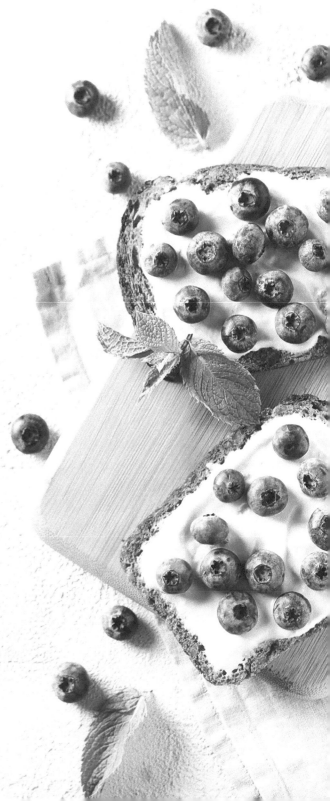

SIMPLY
WHOLESOME

EASY. BALANCED RECIPES FOR A HEALTH CONSCIOUS LIFESTYLE

SHANI ROSENBAUM

a healthy outside
STARTS FROM THE INSIDE

Hi, for those of you who don't know me, I'm Shani from Shape by Shani, a personal training studio in Baltimore, where I live. My philosophy is all about empowerment, helping people become physically, mentally, and emotionally healthy through physical fitness. How does that work?

When you build these skills, your self-confidence will soar. You will discover strengths within yourself that you didn't know existed, and in doing so you'll be able to accomplish personal goals outside the fitness world.

But back to this cookbook. I decided to create this collection of recipes after realizing I was spending too much time scrolling on my Instagram to find all my favorite recipes. I love graphic design, and I decided to hop on Canva and make a cookbook for myself and for you guys. The recipes in here are quick and easy. For me, spending hours on a recipe and standing long hours in the kitchen doesn't work. I love my kitchen, don't get me wrong, but cooking wise, the shorter the better. You'll find that you have most of the ingredients for the recipes in this book sitting right in your pantry, fridge or spice cabinets. And trust me, these recipes are delicious! I am a very picky eater, and I find that I do not like most veggies, so getting those nutrients in was tricky. I made it work by creating yummy soups and salads. I found that the more I played around with spices, the more I actually started to like veggies. Wait, don't get too excited; some veggies; not all. Yes, miracles do happen sometimes.

As the title says above, as great as we can make ourselves look on the outside, unless it starts from the inside, it won't do us much good. Physically, we need to balance proper self-care with healthy nutrition, exercise, fresh air, and sleep in order to feel our best.

Anyways, I hope you enjoy making these simple, easy, and balanced meals as a way to make nutrition a fun and stress-free part of your life.

xoxo, shan

Grocery & Shopping List

In this cookbook there are ingredients listed, and this page will tell you which products to get that are most beneficial for our bodies. These are the products I use for myself and what I tell my clients to get as well. Most of these products can be bought on Amazon at a low cost.

- High-Powered blender for Smoothies: Ninja, Vitamix, or Oster.
- Food scale
- Food processor
- Air fryer
- Protein powder—I use whey from Nutrabio.com
- Unsweetened almond milk—I use Blue Diamond; you can get flavored or unflavored.
- Smart balance butter—make sure you get the pareve one.
- Greek yogurt—aim for the plain ones; if you can't stand those, like me, you can get the 100-calorie Greek yogurts; use the vanilla flavor; these come in Cholov Yisroel too.
- Trader Joe's Everything But the Bagel seasoning-no explanation needed! I use this spice on everything!
- Nutritional yeast—this can be sprinkled on all kinds of veggies.
- Peanut butter—<u>this is important</u>-make sure the ingredients <u>only</u> list peanuts, nothing else, no sugar, salt, oil, etc; this also goes for almond and cashew butter.
- PB2—this is an alternative to peanut butter; it's a powder made out of peanuts. It's way lower in calories than regular peanut butter, and can be added to smoothies or oatmeal.
- Unsweetened apple sauce pouches—these are a great low-calorie, low-sugar snack; they come in other flavors as well, like strawberry and blueberry.
- Vegetable and chicken broth—I use the low-sodium Imagine brand
- Salad dressing—my personal favorite is the Saladmate brand; use 1 tbsp. of the light version; It will coat your whole salad and still be enough. (if you don't have access to that brand, you can make your own and use 1 tbsp. of it)
- Beet chips—an excellent topping for salads; I use the Rhythm Superfoods brand from Amazon

Nutrition and Fitness Guidelines

- Eat unprocessed foods, such as oats and blueberries, not a blueberry muffin! Look for simple, natural ingredients, especially ones that include the word "whole." The ingredients that are listed first make up the largest part of the product. (You don't want the first ingredient to be sugar!)

- Simplify your meals—every meal should include fruits, grains, vegetables, and protein.

- Eat slower and avoid distractions, such as watching TV, talking on the phone, etc.

- Be mindful of your body. Eat when you are hungry. Stop when you are full. Be aware of hunger cues.

- Stay hydrated by drinking your daily water amount. Take your weight and divide it in half—that's how many ounces of water you should aim for a day.

- Amp up your veggies. Eat the rainbow.

- According to USDA guidelines, try to make at least half of your grains whole. This can include whole wheat products.

- Aim for at least 25 grams of fiber a day. Examples are raspberries, split peas, lentils, beans, broccoli, apples and barley.

- Aim for **10,000+ steps** a day.

- Aim for 150-300 minutes (2.5 hours) of moderate-intensity or 75-150 minutes (1 hour and 15 minutes) of high- intensity exercise a week.

TABLE OF CONTENTS

breakfast   p. 9

smoothies   p. 31

snacks   p. 61

soups & side dishes   p. 73

dinners   p. 113

dessert   p. 143

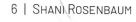

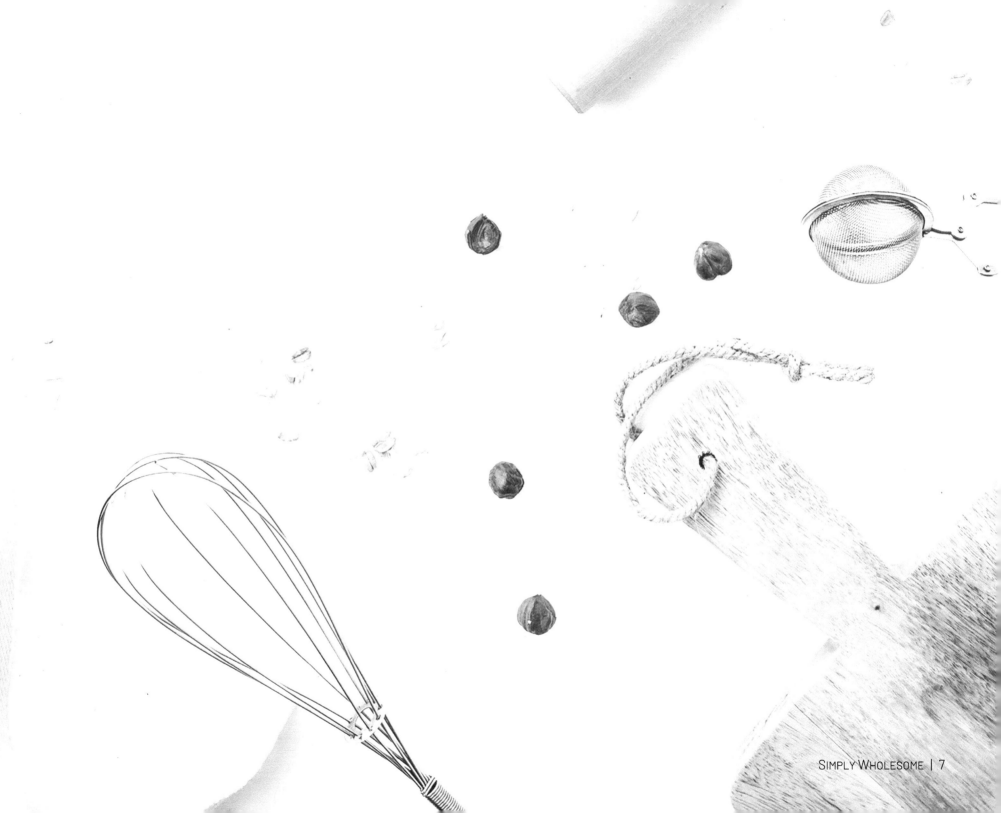

say good morning to your body

- egg omelet
- hot cocoa
- oatmeal
- granola
- blueberry protein muffin

- protein pancakes
- mini pancakes
- iced coffee
- cottage cheese
- matcha

a good breakfast

IS THE START OF A GOOD DAY

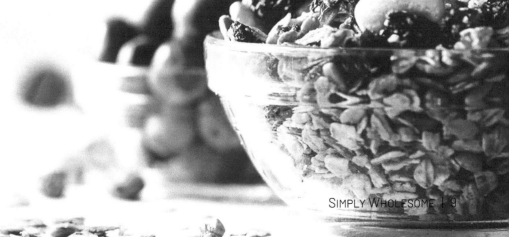

EGG OMELET

My go-to breakfast every morning. Takes less than 5 minutes, and it gives me 25 grams of protein!!

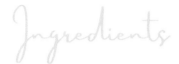

Ingredients

- 1 cup egg whites
- 1 egg yolk
- Avocado/coconut/olive oil spray
- Salt and pepper, to taste
- Mushrooms (optional)
- Onions (optional)
- Spinach (optional)

Spray oil onto non-stick frying pan.

Pour egg whites and egg yolk into pan.

Add toppings of your choice. Scramble.

Sprinkle salt and pepper.

Serve immediately.

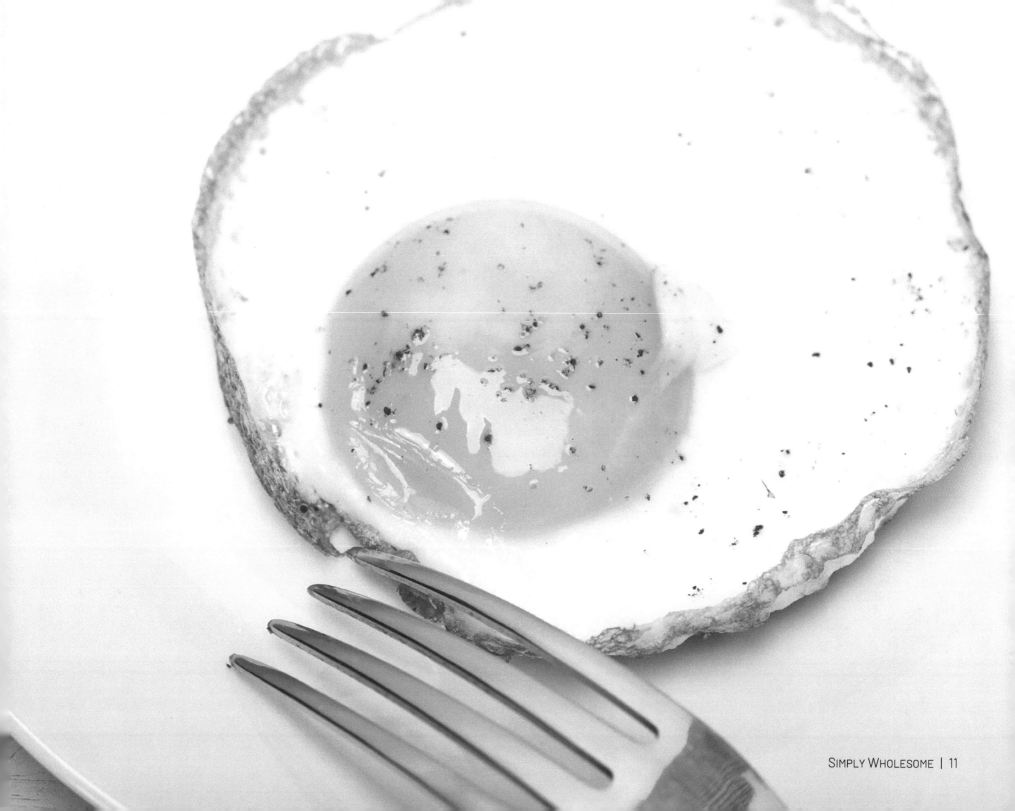

HOT COCOA

- 2 tbsp. unsweetened cocoa powder
- 2 tbsp. stevia
- 1 cup unsweetened almond milk
- 1/8 tsp. vanilla extract
- Pinch of salt
- 1 cup water

Whisk together the cocoa powder, stevia, almond milk, vanilla extract, salt, and water in a microwave-safe bowl.
Microwave hot cocoa for about 1 minute or until it is piping hot.
Stir until all powder is dissolved and fully blended.

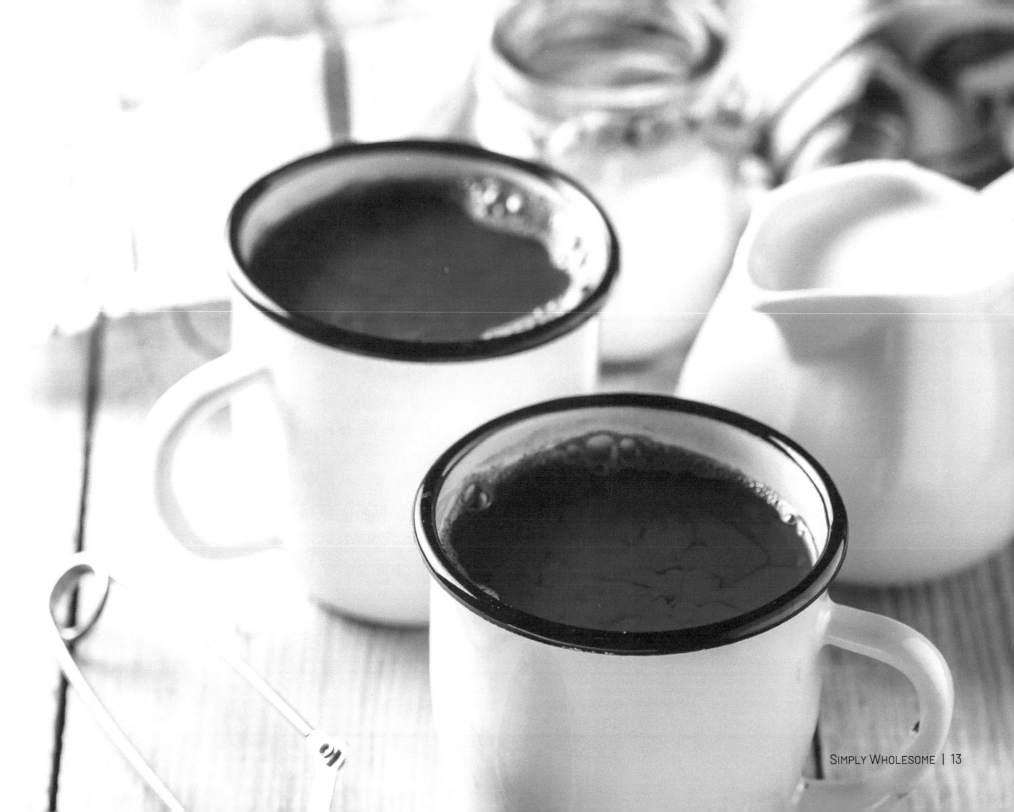

HEART-HEALTHY OATMEAL

Oatmeal is so good for you. It's got tons of fiber and minerals, leaving you full and satiated. An added plus that it's one of the world's healthiest grains and is gluten free. #winwin

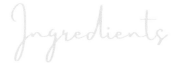

Ingredients

- 1/2 cup oats
- 1/2 cup unsweetened almond milk
- 1/2 cup water
- Pinch salt

In a small saucepan, bring the water and milk to a boil. Reduce the heat to low and pour in the oats. Cook, stirring occasionally, until the oats are soft and have absorbed most of the liquid, about 5 minutes. Remove from the heat, cover, and let stand for 2-3 minutes.

Now for the fun part: the toppings! Feel free to choose some of these. Not all!

- Any fruit—berries work well, also banana slices
- Granola—use my recipe on p. 16. Add 1-2 tbsp.
- Protein powder—1 scoop
- Nuts—use 1 tbsp.
- Drizzle peanut butter—1 tsp.
- Spices—vanilla, cinnamon, nutmeg
- Honey—just a drizzle
- Chia seeds

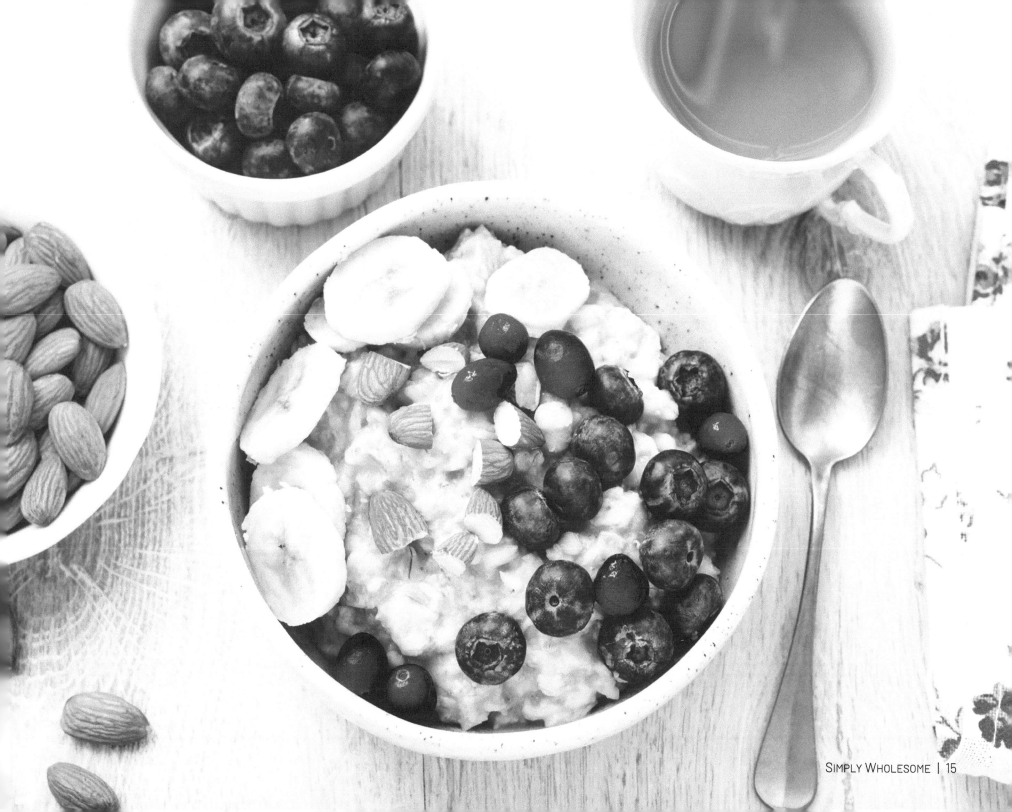

GRANOLA

Now you can make your own granola instead of the store bought ones.

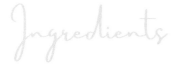

- 2 cups walnuts, chopped
- 1/2 cup dried craisins, optional
- 1/4 cup pumpkin seeds
- 3 tbsp. sunflower seeds
- 3 tbsp. flax seeds
- 3 tbsp. olive or coconut oil
- 2 tbsp. maple syrup
- 1 tbsp. pure vanilla extract
- 1 tbsp. ground cinnamon
- 2 tsp. pumpkin spice
- 1 tsp. sea salt

Preheat oven to 300 °F and line a baking sheet with parchment paper.

Combine all ingredients and stir until well coated. Spread mixture out.

Bake for 15-17 minutes.

Add granola to your yogurts, oatmeal, or as a fruit topping.

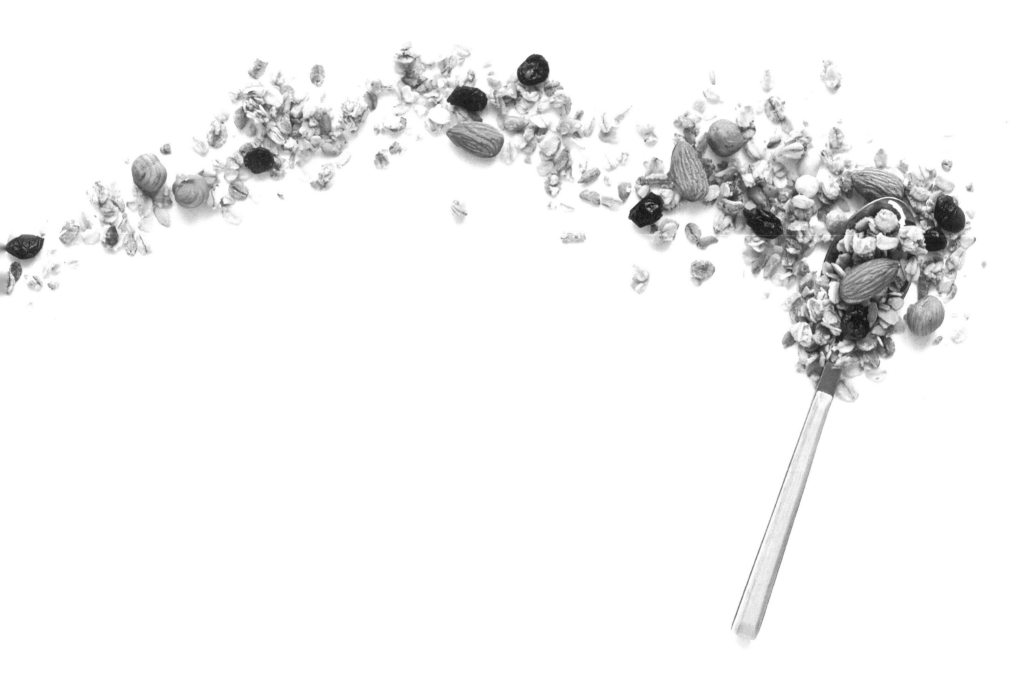

BLUEBERRY PROTEIN MUFFINS

Your kids will love these! I mean, who doesn't love muffins, right? These are just like the Dunkin' ones. Okay, maybe I'm exaggerating, but they really are delicious.

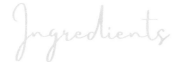

Ingredients

- 3/4 cup vanilla protein powder
- 1 tbsp. baking powder
- 1 cup oat flour
- 2 large eggs, whisked
- 1/4 cup honey
- 1 cup banana
- 3/4 cup water
- Fresh blueberries

Preheat oven to 350 °F. Grease an 8-count muffin tin. Add dry ingredients and mix. Add eggs, banana, honey, and water and mix until well combined. Sprinkle the blueberries into the mix. Don't mix the blueberries in. Bake for 22 minutes.

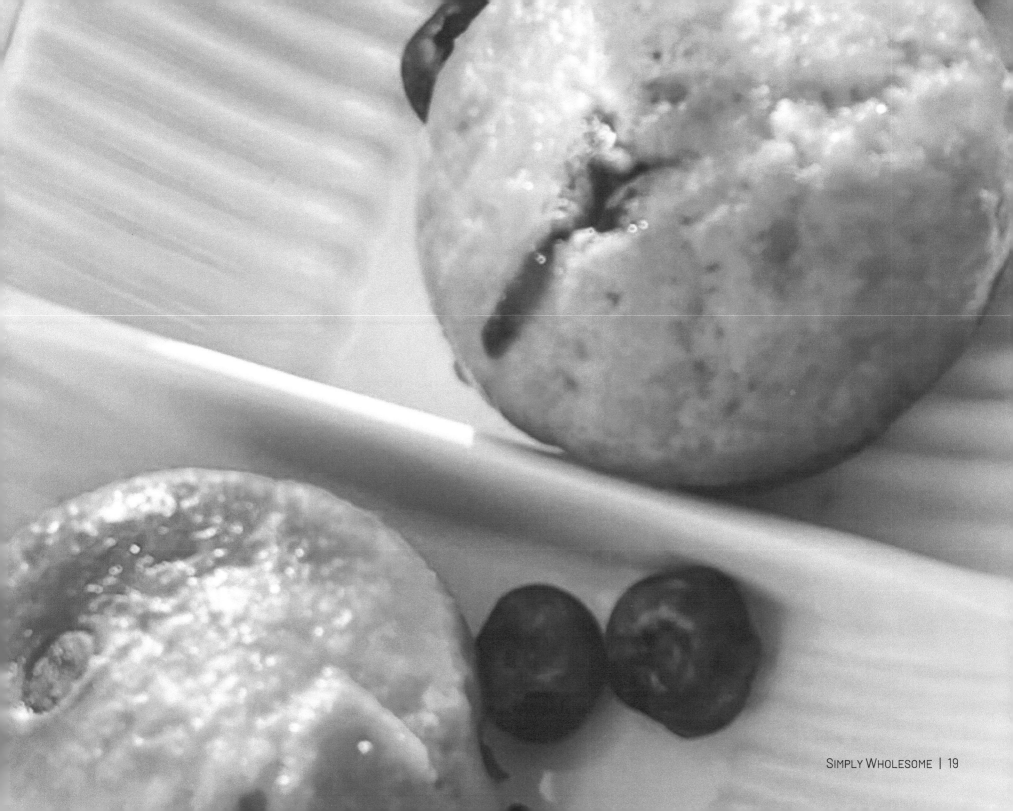

PROTEIN PANCAKES

Who says pancakes are just for kids?

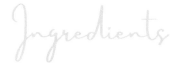

Ingredients

- 1 whole egg
- 2 tbsp. egg whites
- 1 tsp. maple syrup/vanilla + extra for drizzle
- 1 scoop vanilla protein powder
- 1/4 cup unsweetened almond milk
- Top with berries of choice or nuts

Blend ingredients in blender.

Spray pan with olive or avocado oil spray.

Pour a small amount onto pan and flip when lightly brown on sides.

Add 1 tsp. of maple syrup for drizzle and fruit or toppings of choice, optional.

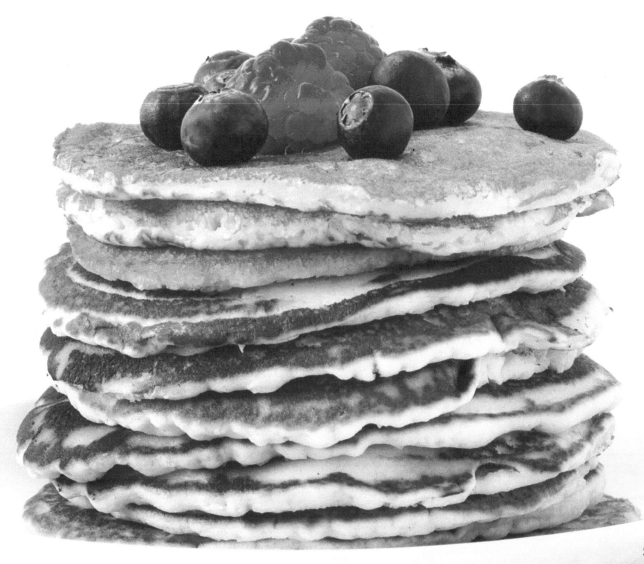

MINI PANCAKES

Aren't these cute?

- 1 cup oats
- 1 cup egg whites
- 1 cup cottage cheese

Blend all ingredients in a blender.

Measure out 1 tbsp. in the pan.

Cook until light brown.

I used PAM olive oil spray and 1 tbsp. coconut oil.

Feel free to top with fresh fruit.

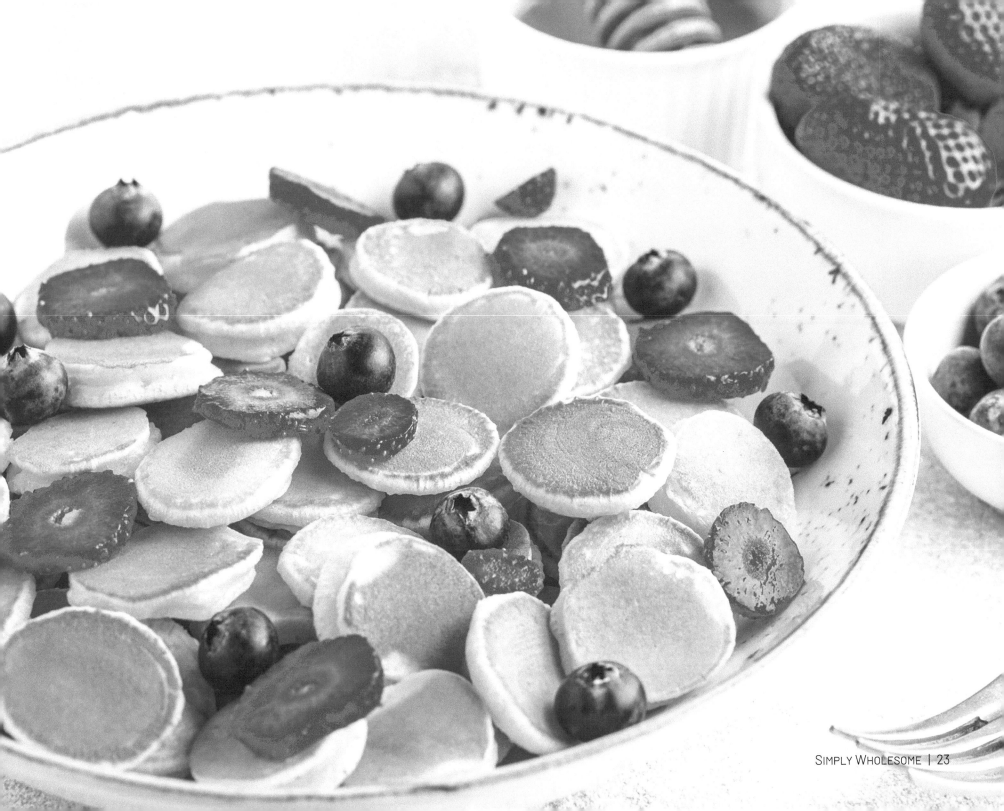

ICED COFFEE

Move over Starbucks-Shape by Shani's iced coffee rules!
But not too far away Starbucks, because I love you.

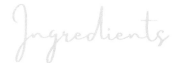

Ingredients

- 1 cup unsweetened almond milk
- 1 scoop vanilla protein powder
- 1 tbsp. decaf coffee mixed with hot water
- 2 tbsp. PB2
- 1 tbsp. sugar-free hazelnut creamer (optional)
- Ice

Dissolve coffee with hot water in a separate cup.

Add coffee mixture to blender.

Add remaining ingredients.

Blend.

Add ice and blend again.

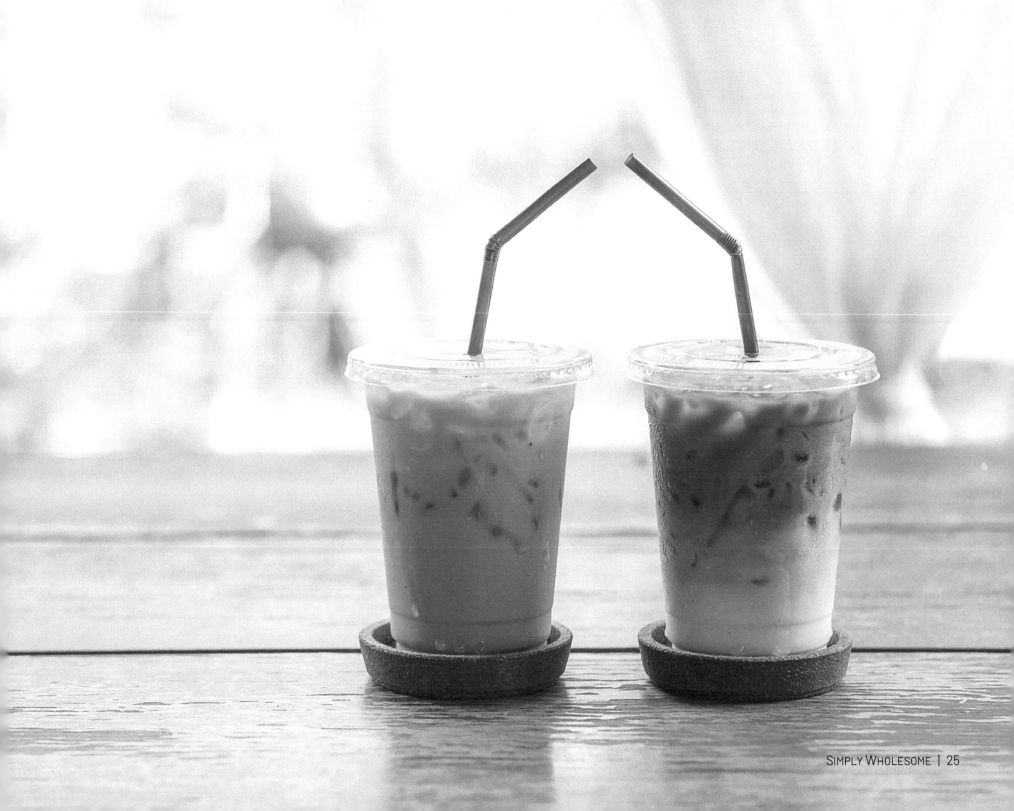

COTTAGE CHEESE WITH TOPPINGS

Cottage cheese is an excellent source of protein.

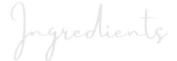

- 1/2 cup of cottage cheese
- 1 tsp. each of sunflower seeds, pomegranate seeds, walnuts and almonds + drizzle of honey

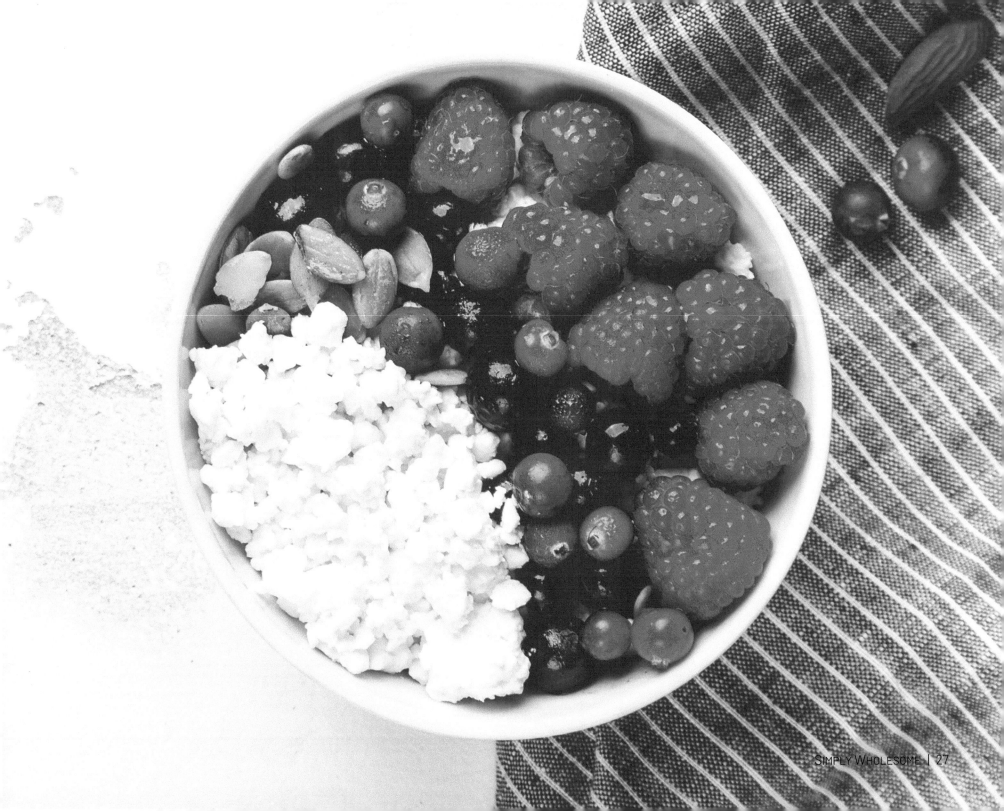

MATCHA DRINK

For those of you who are unfamiliar with matcha, it is a powdered green tea and is energizing like coffee, without the crash afterward

---

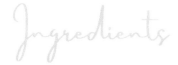

- 1/2 cup unsweetened almond milk
- 1/2 tsp. matcha powder
- 1/2 tsp. pure maple syrup or honey

Heat the milk over medium heat and bring to a simmer.
Pour hot milk and powder into blender, adding in your choice of sweetener.
Blend on high speed for 20 seconds.
Serve warm.

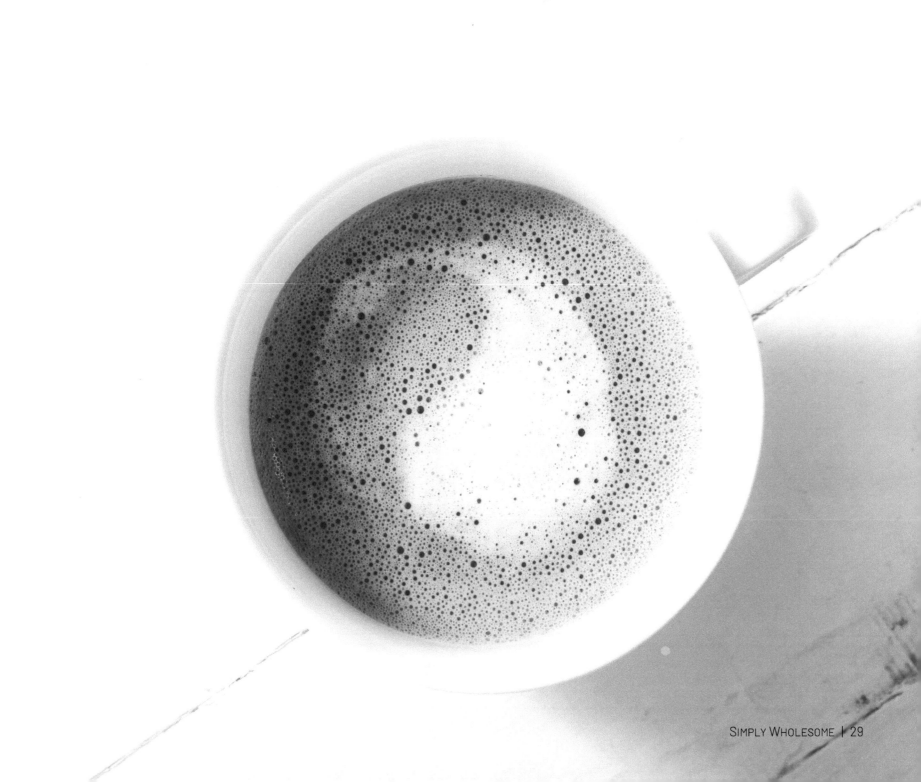

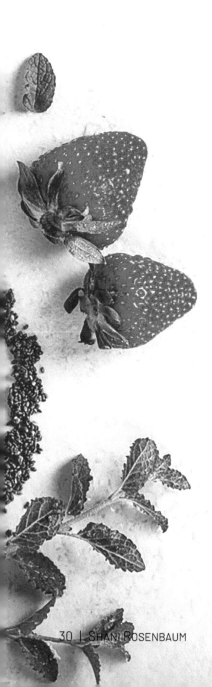

- raspberry protein shake
- blueberry protein shake
- kale smoothie bowl
- strawberry kiwi shake
- vanilla protein shake
- start your day fresh
- healthy green smoothie

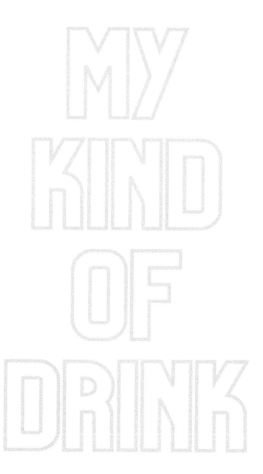

MY KIND OF DRINK

- peanut butter protein shake
- yogurt fruit bowl
- chocolate raspberry shake
- beet smoothie bowl
- you're such a smoothie!
- green shake
- feel better soon!

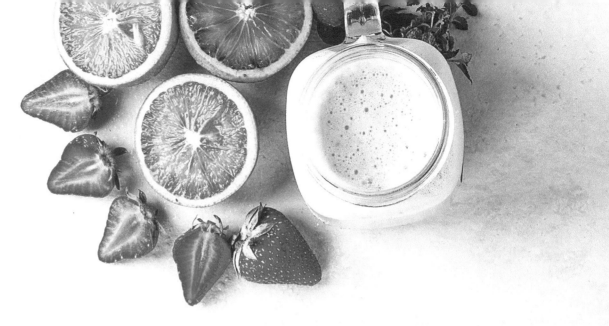

SMOOTHIES

my kind of drink

RASPBERRY SMOOTHIE

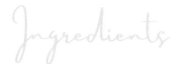

- 3/4 cup unsweetened almond milk
- 2 scoops vanilla protein powder
- 1 container plain Greek yogurt
- 1 cup raspberries
- 2 tsp. honey (optional for sweetness)

Blend with a high-speed blender and bon appétit

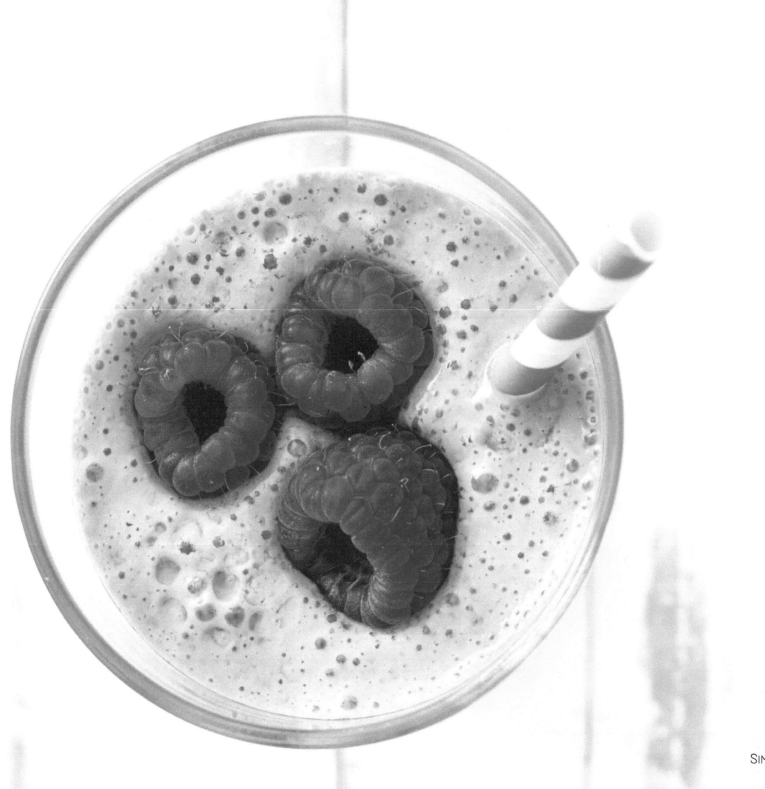

BLUEBERRY SMOOTHIE

Ingredients

- 1 cup blueberries
- 1 container vanilla Greek yogurt (100 calories)
- 1 cup unsweetened almond milk
- Ice

Blend and bon appétit

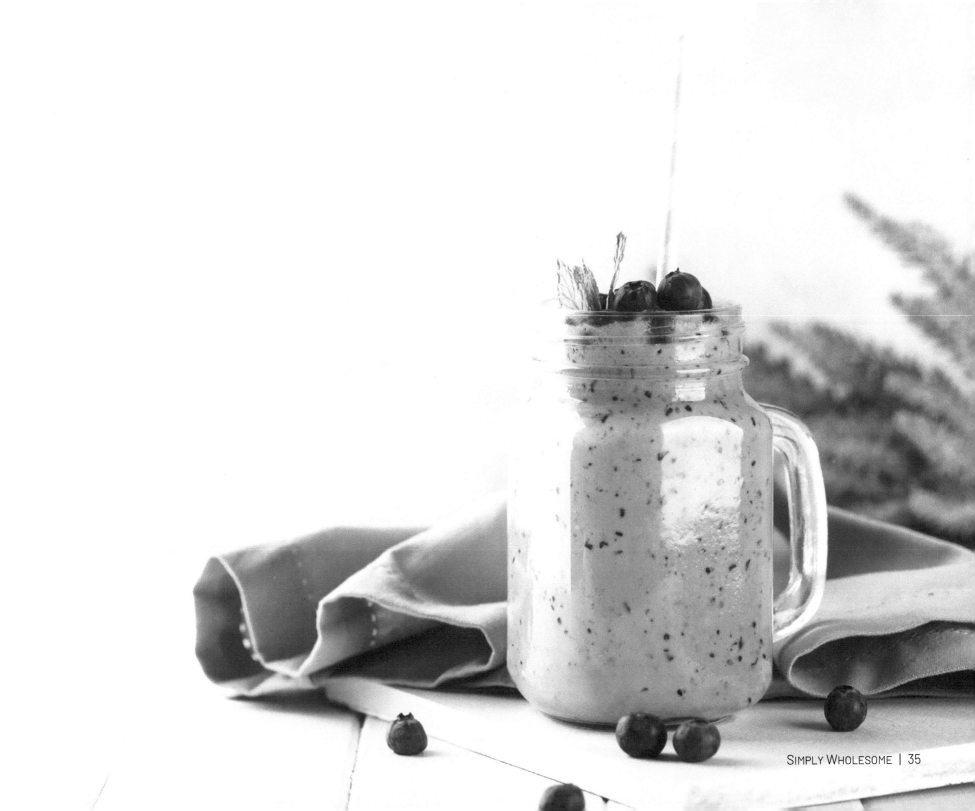

KALE SMOOTHIE BOWL WITH TOPPINGS

Feel free to substitute the kale with spinach leaves.
Flax seeds are a good source of Omega-3 and have both soluble and insoluble fibers

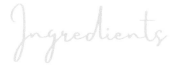

- 2 cups kale
- 1 banana, frozen
- 1 tbsp. honey
- 1/2 cup Greek yogurt
- 1 tbsp. almond butter
- 1 tsp. vanilla
- 1/2 cup coconut water
- 2 tbsp. flax seeds
- 1 scoop vanilla whey protein powder

Mix all ingredients in a blender. Make sure it's mixed very well.

Add your favorite toppings: banana, pomegranate seeds, chia seeds, kiwi, or pineapple chunks.

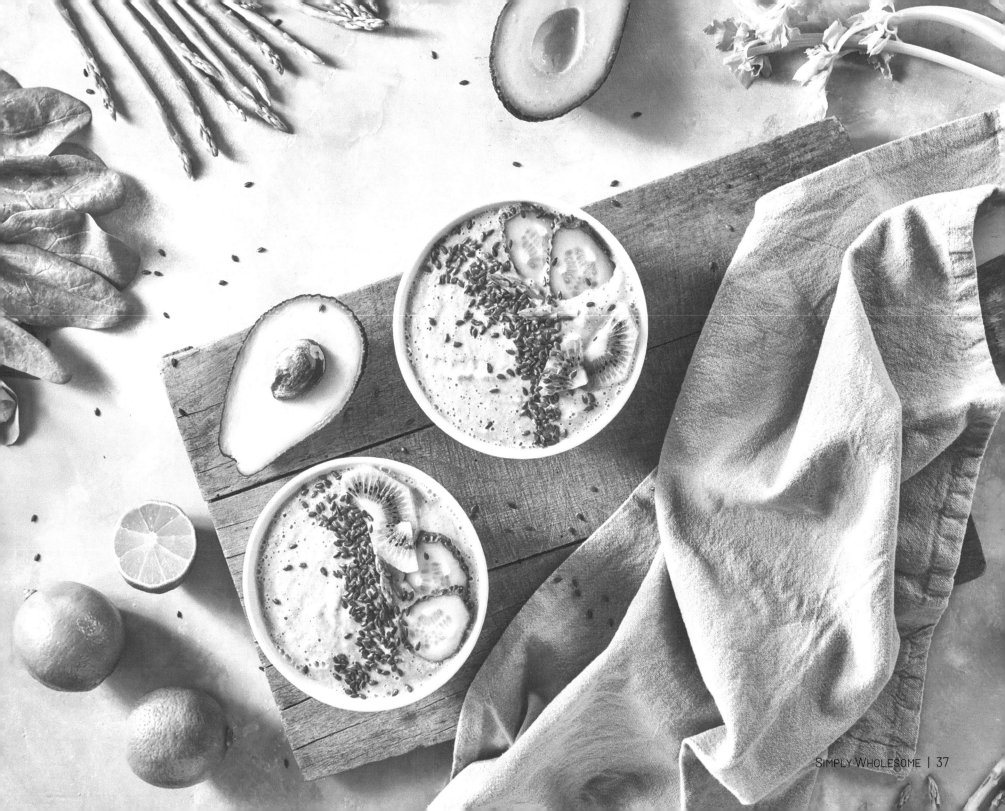

STRAWBERRY KIWI SMOOTHIE

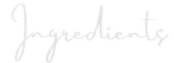

- 6 strawberries
- 3 kiwis
- 1 container of vanilla Greek yogurt (100 calories)
- 1 cup unsweetened almond milk

Blend and bon appétit

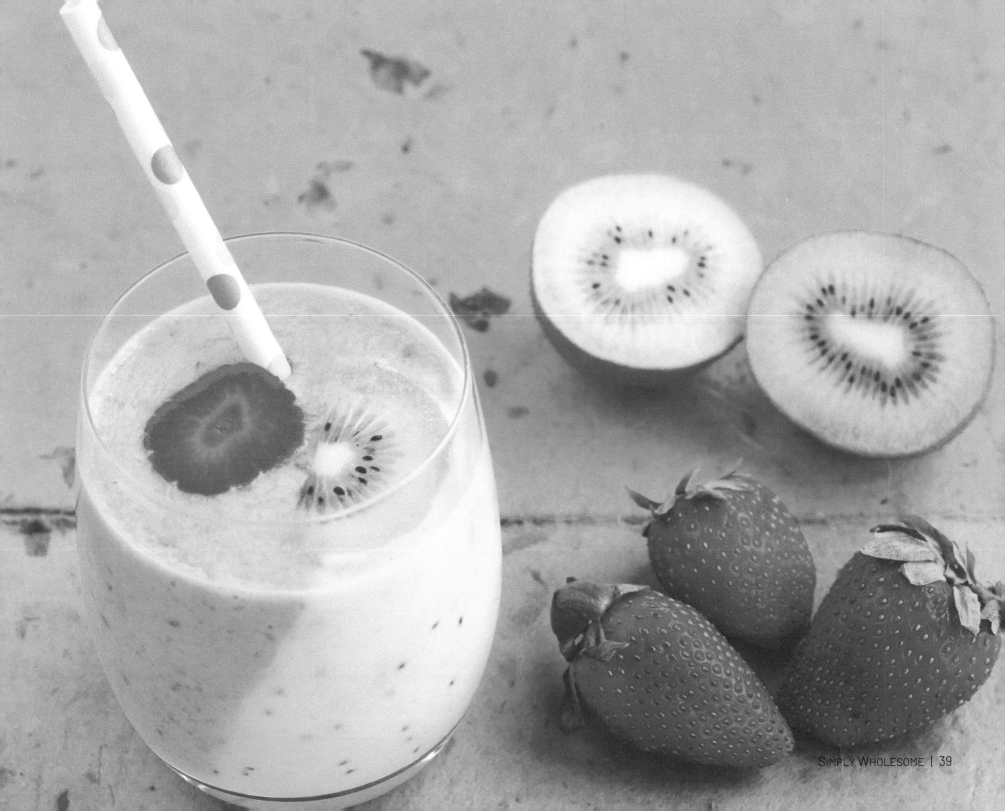

VANILLA PROTEIN SHAKE

- 1 vanilla Greek yogurt (100 calories)
- 1/2 cup unsweetened almond milk
- 1 tbsp. vanilla
- 1 scoop vanilla protein powder
- Ice

Blend. The chocolate is for design purposes only

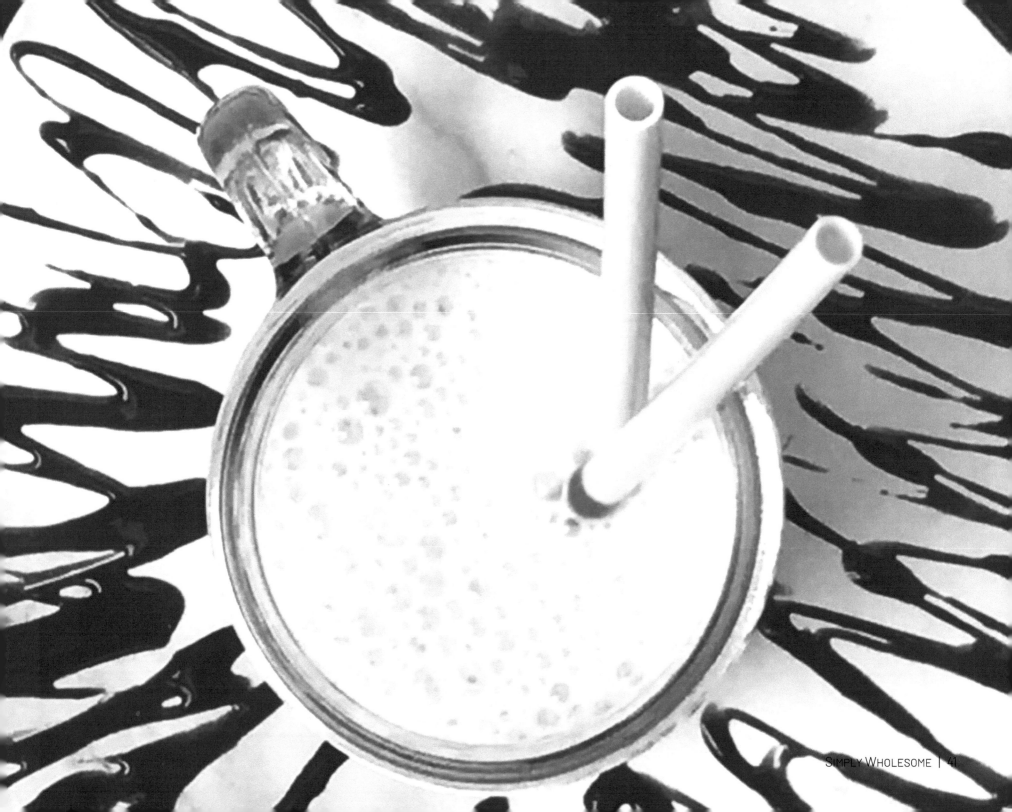

START YOUR DAY FRESH

A full meal right here: you got your protein, healthy fat, and carbs. You are ready to take on the day!

Ingredients

- 1/2 cup strawberries
- 1 cup blueberries
- 1 container of vanilla Greek yogurt (100 calories)
- 1 package almonds (100 calories)
- 1/2 banana (optional)
- 1 cup unsweetened almond milk

Blend and drink immediately.

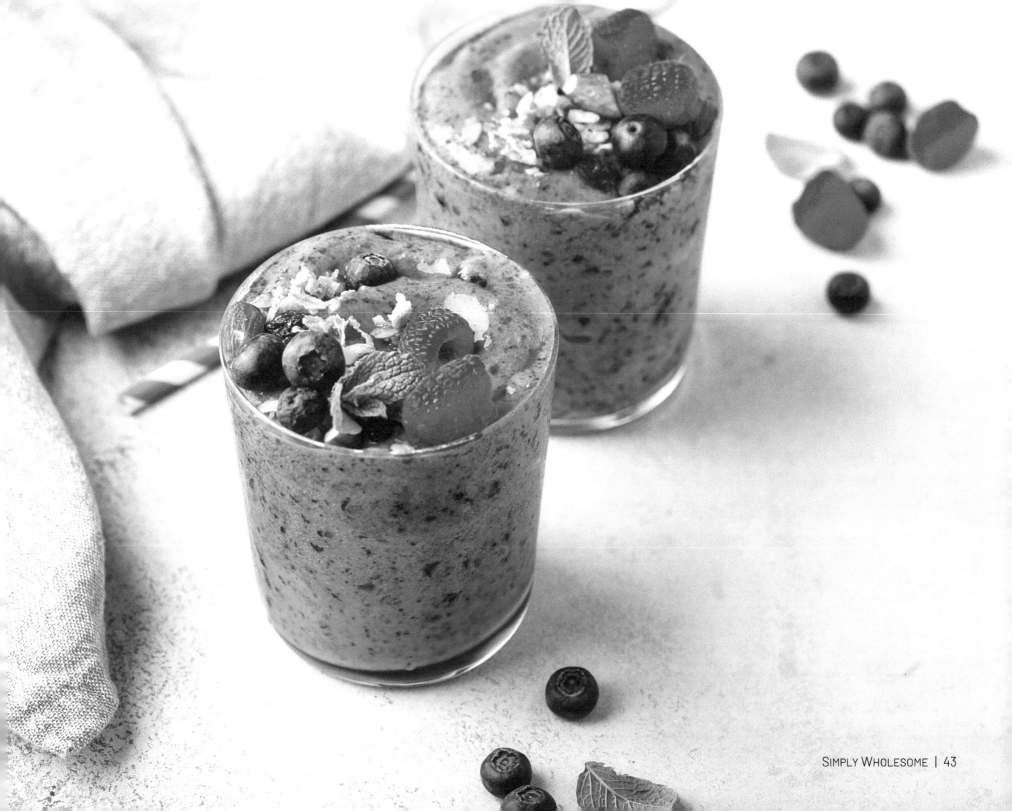

HEALTHY GREEN SMOOTHIE

I was introduced to a "green" smoothie with this recipe, from a friend of mine. She assured me I wouldn't taste the kale or the avocado, which I don't like. I decided to trust her and it was love at first sight. From then on, I wasn't scared of green smoothies anymore and now they are a part of my life.

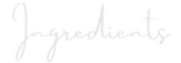

Ingredients

- A handful of power greens (Trader Joe's has it)
- 1 green apple
- 1 banana
- handful of frozen pineapple
- 1/2 avocado
- 1 lime (use fresh lime, but juice it)
- 1 cup unsweetened almond milk
- water
- ice

Put all ingredients into the blender. Fill the blender with water until it reaches the top.

Blend very well. Drink immediately

It is very important when you are making green smoothies, that your ingredients are extremely fresh. All it takes is one bad avocado, and the smoothie is for the garbage.

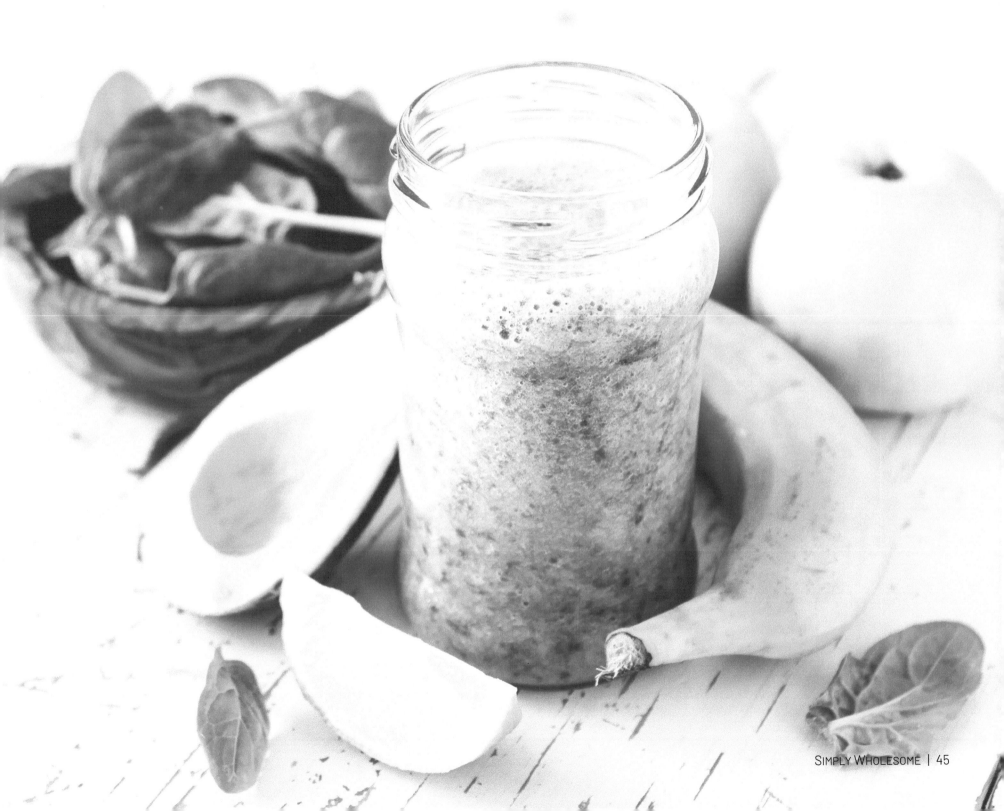

PEANUT BUTTER PROTEIN SMOOTHIE

Make sure your peanut butter only has peanuts listed in the ingredient section.
No oil, sugar, or anything else should be listed. The same goes for almond or cashew butter.

Ingredients

- 1 cup unsweetened almond milk
- 1 scoop vanilla protein powder
- 1 tsp. peanut butter or 2 tbsp. PB2
- Ice

Blend and drink up!

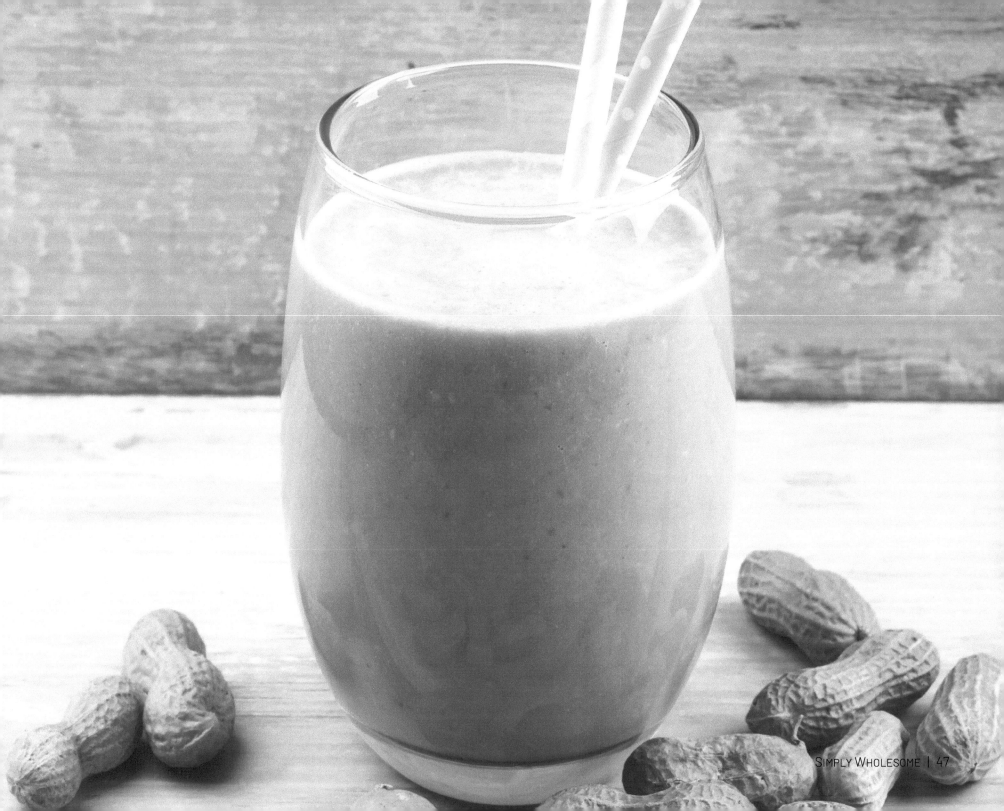

YOGURT FRUIT BOWL

Don't be fooled by the "açai" bowls at restaurants, thinking oh it's mostly fruit, so it's healthy!
Most of the time the quantities are in very large amounts, bumping the calories way up.
The ingredients may be healthy, but quantity matters too. Here you can make your own "fruit bowl" and have control
over the amount of fruit and toppings you are adding in, thereby making it a low-calorie, high-protein meal.

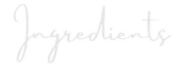

- 2 100-calorie vanilla Greek yogurts
- 1 tbsp. pomegranate seeds
- 1 tbsp. sliced almonds
- 1 tbsp. sunflower seeds
- 1/2 banana, cut into cubes

Take out a bowl and first put in the yogurt, then add the toppings afterwards.

Enjoy!

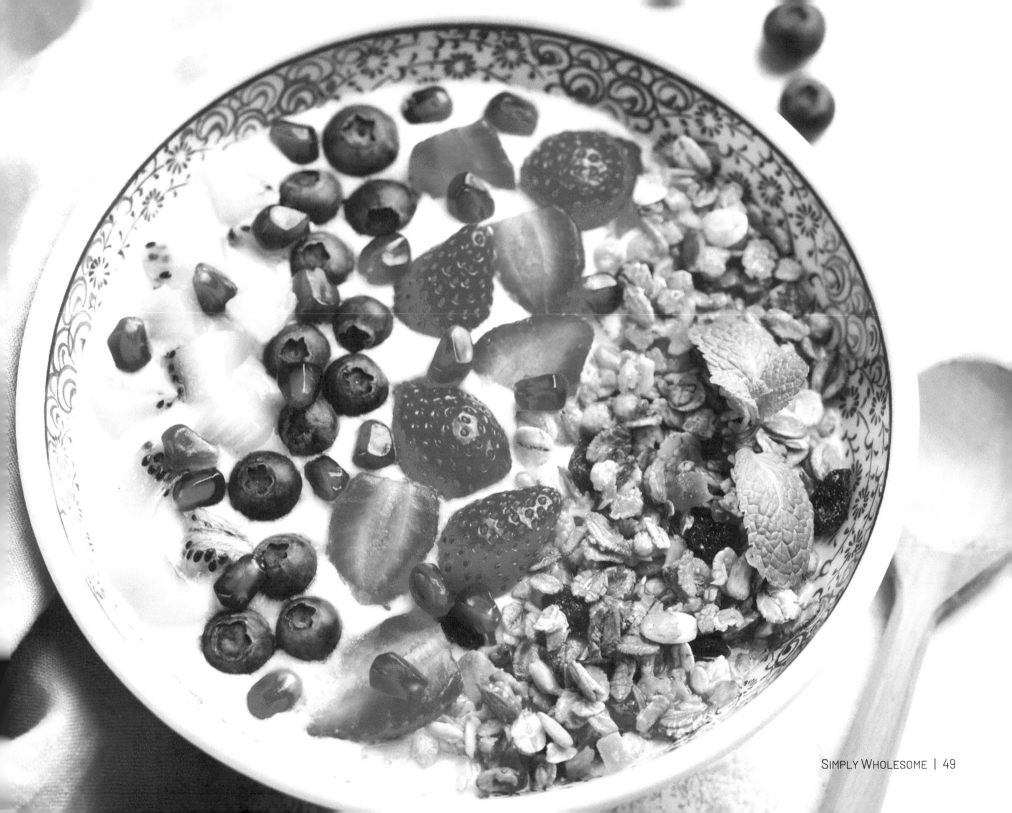

CHOCOLATE RASPBERRY PROTEIN SHAKE

Don't worry, you won't taste the cauliflower at all! Just thought I'd sneak in a good source of fiber for you.
The flax seeds can easily be swapped with chia seeds, another good source of fiber.
See how I take care of you guys?

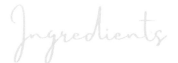

- 1 scoop vanilla protein powder
- 8 oz. unsweetened almond milk
- 1 tbsp. unsweetened cocoa
- 1 tbsp. flax seeds
- 1 small handful frozen cauliflower rice
- 1/2 cup raspberries
- Ice

Using a high-power blender, put in the liquid first and then add the rest of the ingredients. Blend for 30 seconds, and then add ice and blend again.

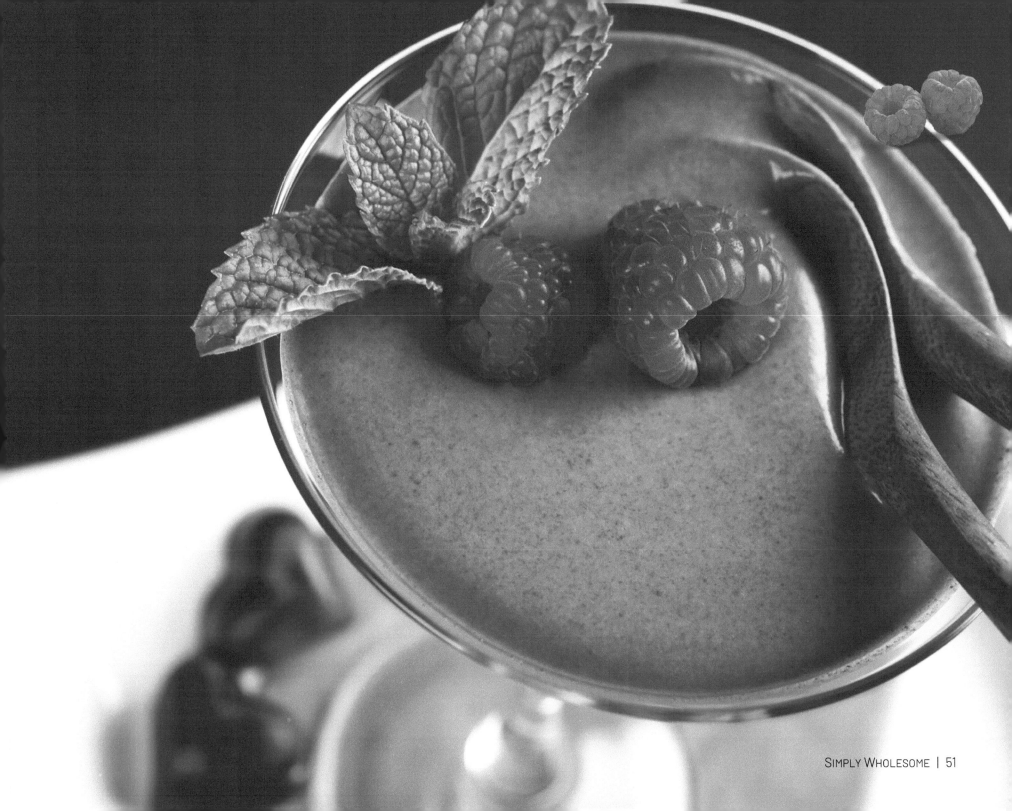

BEET SMOOTHIE BOWL

A good source of fiber, potassium, and healthy fat

Ingredients

- 1 can beets
- 1/2 cup raspberries
- 1/2 avocado
- 1/2 banana
- 1 tbsp. vanilla protein powder
- Ice

Blend until smooth. Add your favorite toppings.

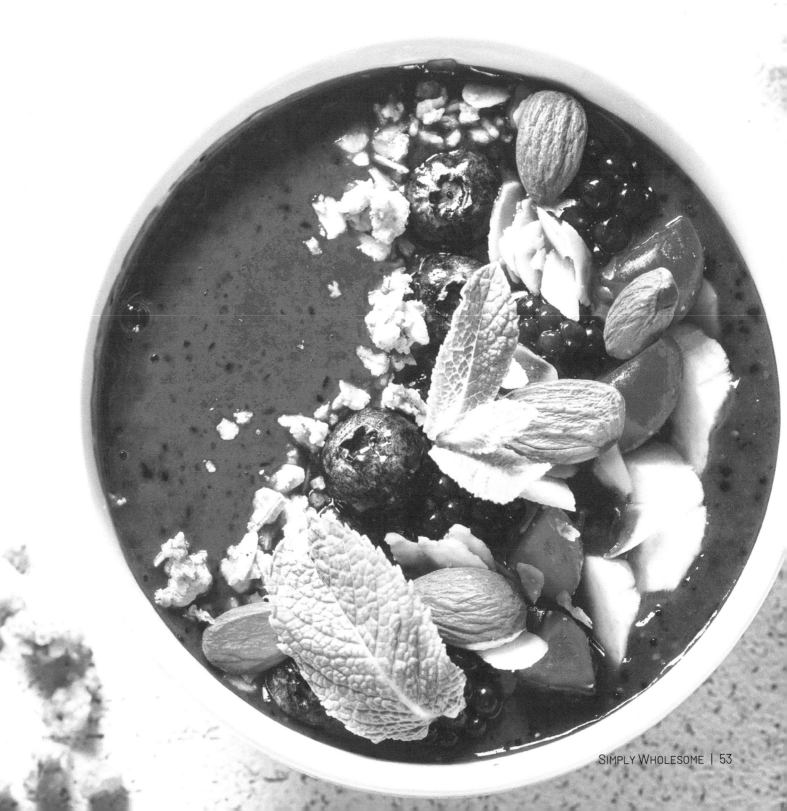

YOU'RE SUCH A SMOOTHIE!

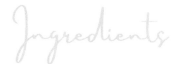

- 6 strawberries
- 3 kiwis
- 1 nectarine
- 1 tbsp. mixed nuts
- 1 container plain Greek yogurt
- 1/2–1 cup unsweetened almond milk, depending on how thick you want it to be.

Blend, using a blender. Add your favorite toppings.

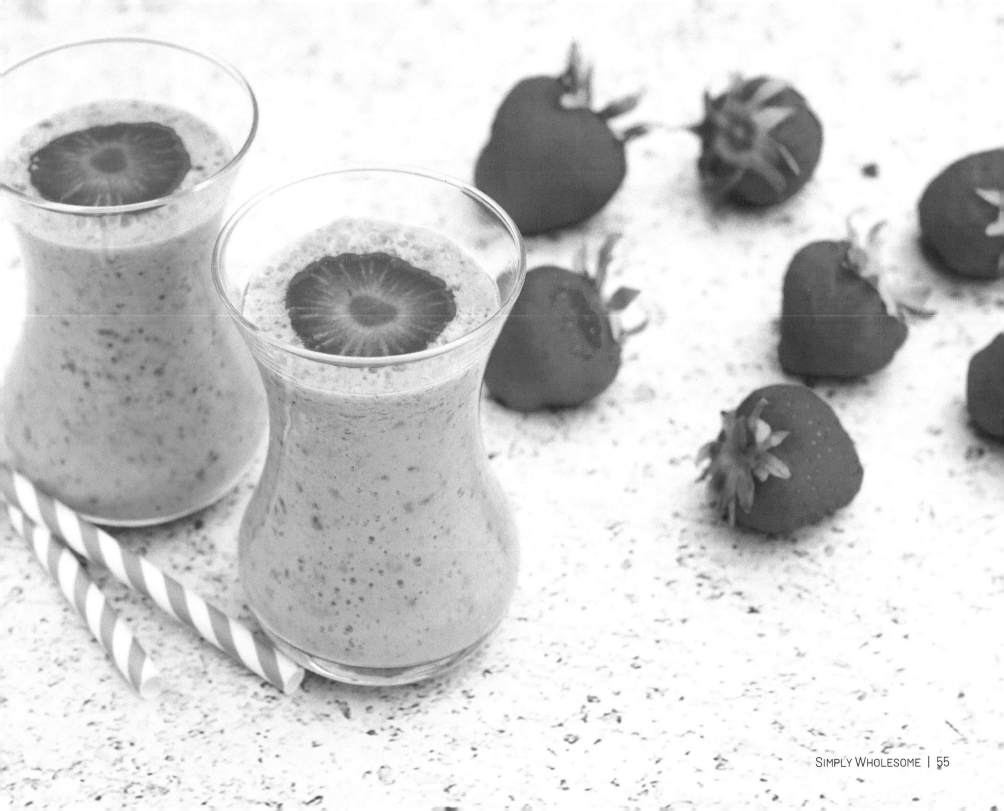

GREEN SMOOTHIE

I assure you, you will not taste the spinach or kale. Just try it!

Ingredients

- 1 handful of spinach or kale
- 1 cup unsweetened almond milk
- 2 kiwis
- 1 green apple
- 1/2 banana
- 1 cup water

Blend with Vitamix or nutribullet.

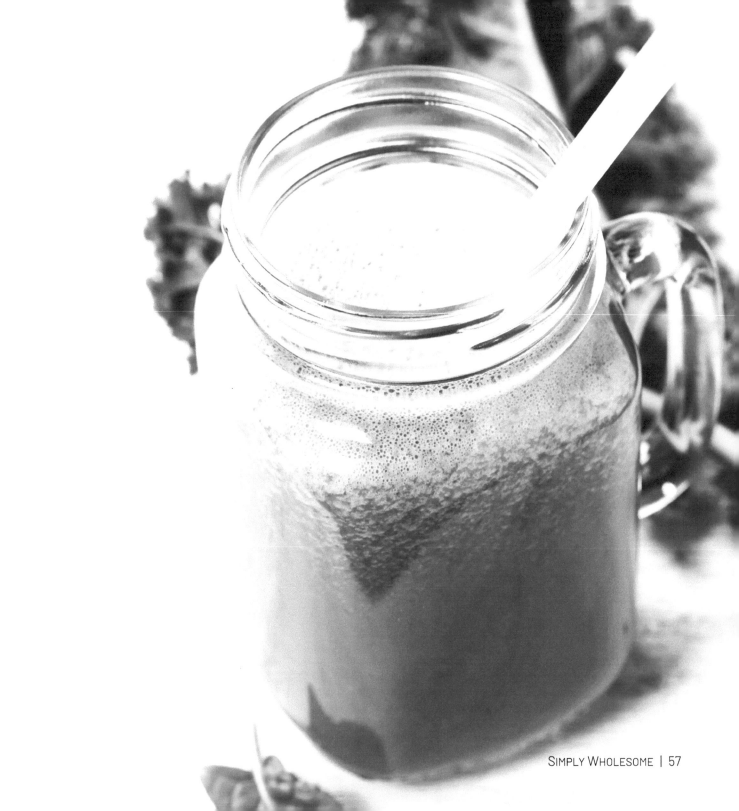

FEEL BETTER SOON SMOOTHIE

*Have a cold? Feeling sick? Turmeric and ginger are known to reduce nausea and improve your immune system.
See how good smoothies are for us?*

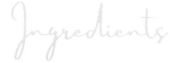

Ingredients

- 1 carrot, chopped
- 1 small orange
- 1/2 banana, frozen
- 1/2 cup frozen mango
- 1/2 cup coconut water
- 1/4 tsp ground turmeric
- 1/4 tsp ground ginger
- Pinch of cayenne pepper
- 1/2 cup ice

Blend everything in a blender.
Add ice and blend. Drink immediately.

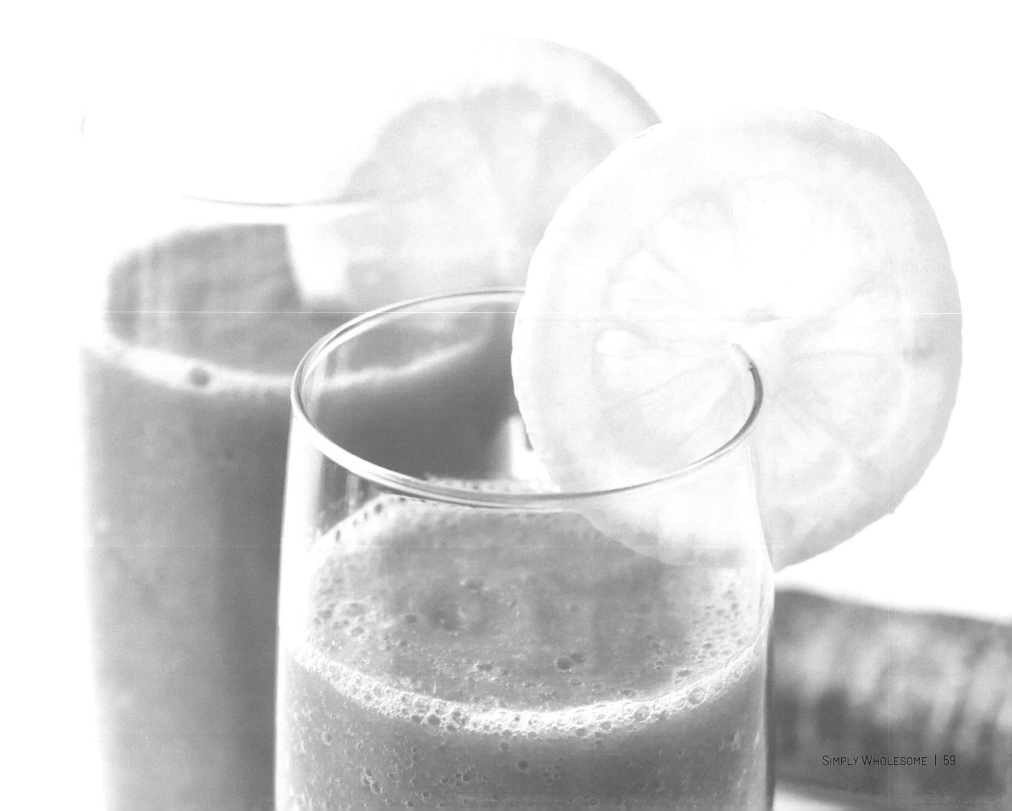

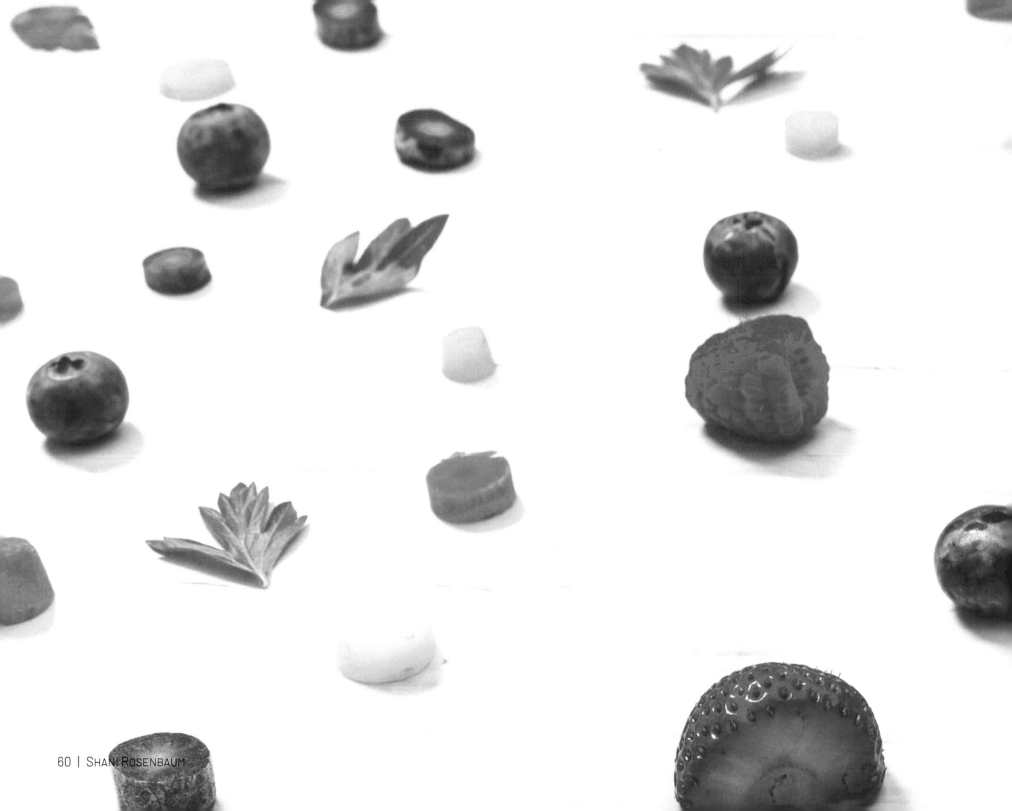

HEALTHY SNACKS FUEL MY *fabulousness*

BANANA MUFFINS WITH PECANS

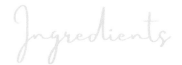

- 3 medium very ripe bananas
- 1 1/4 cups white whole wheat flour
- 3/4 tsp. baking soda
- 1/4 tsp. salt
- 2 tbsp. unsalted butter, softened
- 1/4 cup maple sugar, or brown sugar
- 2 large egg whites
- 1/4 cup pure maple syrup
- 2 tbsp. unsweetened apple sauce
- 1/2 tsp. vanilla extract
- 1/3 cup crushed pecans

Preheat oven to 325 °F. Line a cupcake tin with liners.

Mash bananas in a bowl, set aside.

In a medium bowl, combine flour, baking soda, and salt using a wire whisk. Set aside.

In a large bowl, cream the butter and 1/4 cup sugar with an electric mixer.

Add egg whites, mashed bananas, maple syrup, apple sauce, and vanilla; beat at medium speed until mixed well, scraping down the sides of the bowl.

Add flour mixture, then blend at a low speed until just combined.

Pour the batter into the prepared muffin tin. Spread the pecans evenly over the muffins.

Bake the muffins on the center rack for 30 to 35 minutes, or until a toothpick inserted in the center comes out clean.

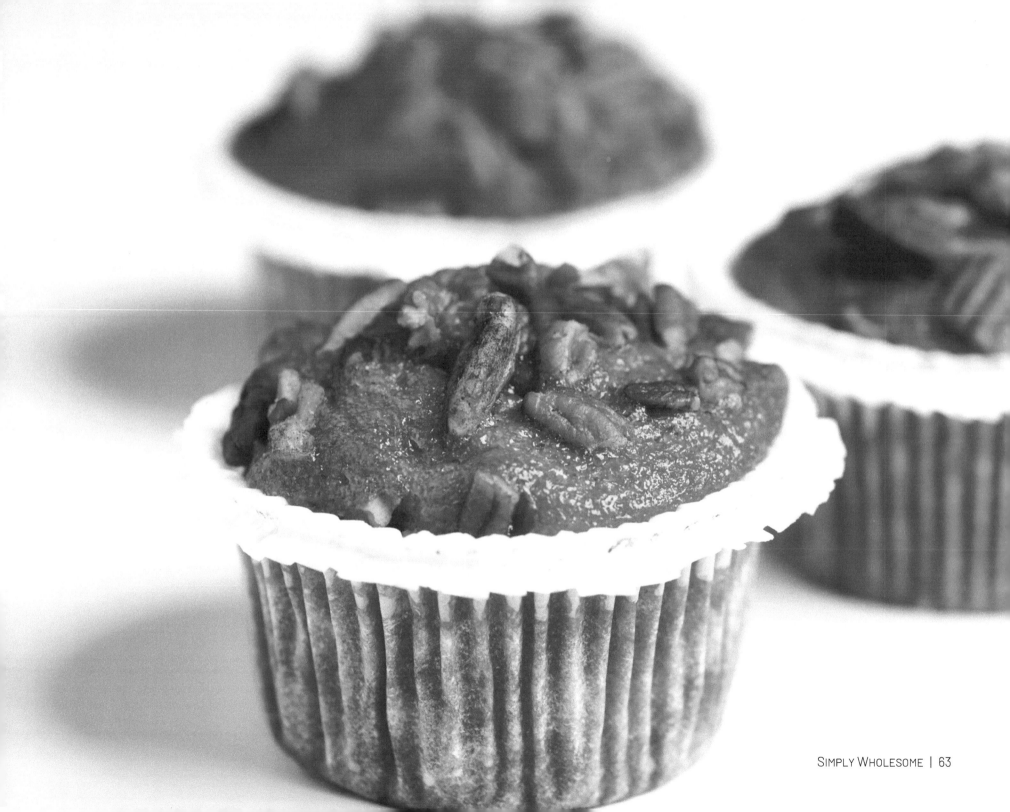

PEANUT BUTTER MINI BANANA MUFFINS

Try not to finish all these in one setting. I challenge you—it will be difficult!

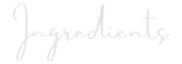

Ingredients

- 1 cup natural peanut butter
- 2 eggs, large
- 2 bananas, mashed
- 1/2 tsp. baking soda
- 1 tsp. vanilla
- mini chocolate chips, (optional)

Blend all ingredients in a blender. Pour into greased mini muffin tins.

Add 2–3 mini chocolate chips on top if you'd like.

Bake at 400 °F for 8 minutes.

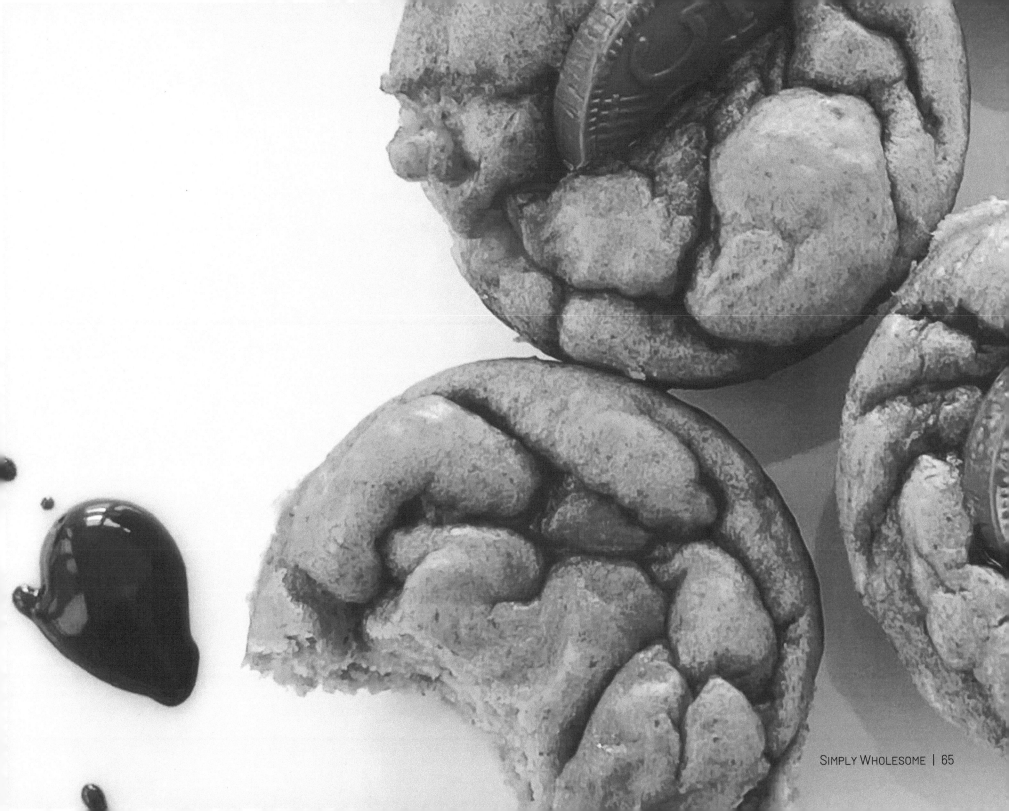

YOGURT BARK

Ingredients

- 100-calorie Chobani vanilla yogurt
- Toppings: sliced almonds, pumpkin seeds, sunflower seeds, strawberries, and pomegranate seeds

Spread the yogurt out on a baking sheet until nice and smooth. Add the toppings and put in the freezer. It is ready when it is frozen—crack it and enjoy.

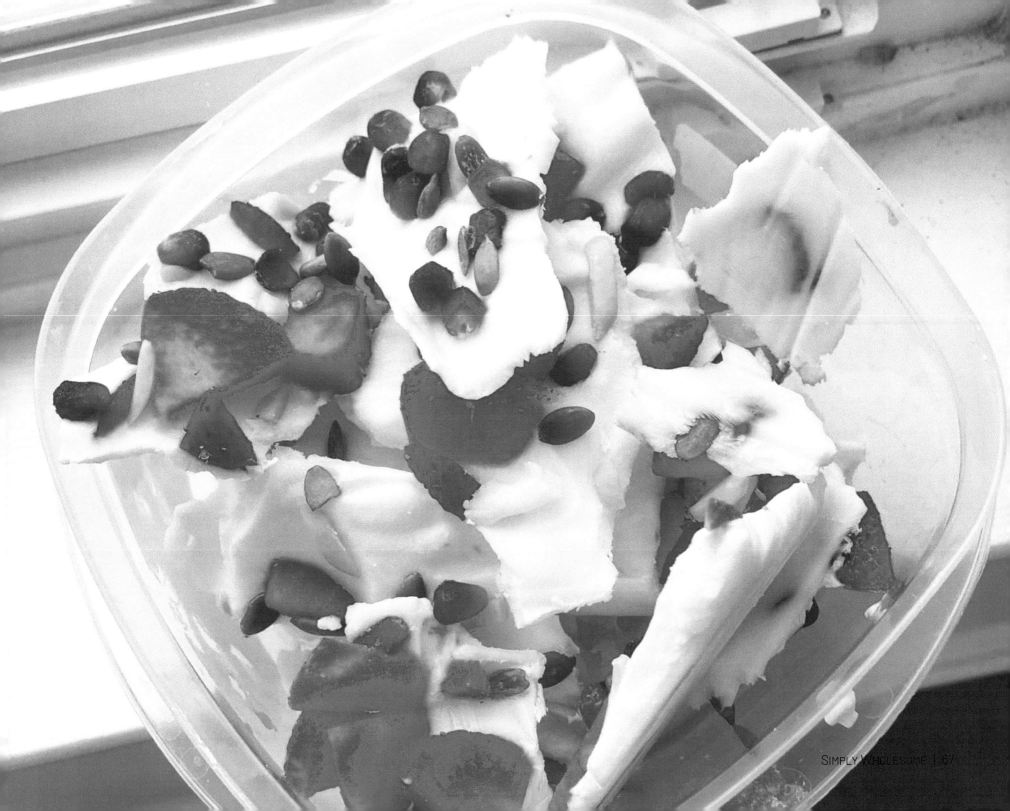

APPLE COOKIES

A great snack: healthy carb + healthy fat = winner! Plus they taste so delicious!

Ingredients

- 1 red apple sliced into thin rings
- 1 tsp. of peanut butter, no salt
- Mini chocolate chips (optional)

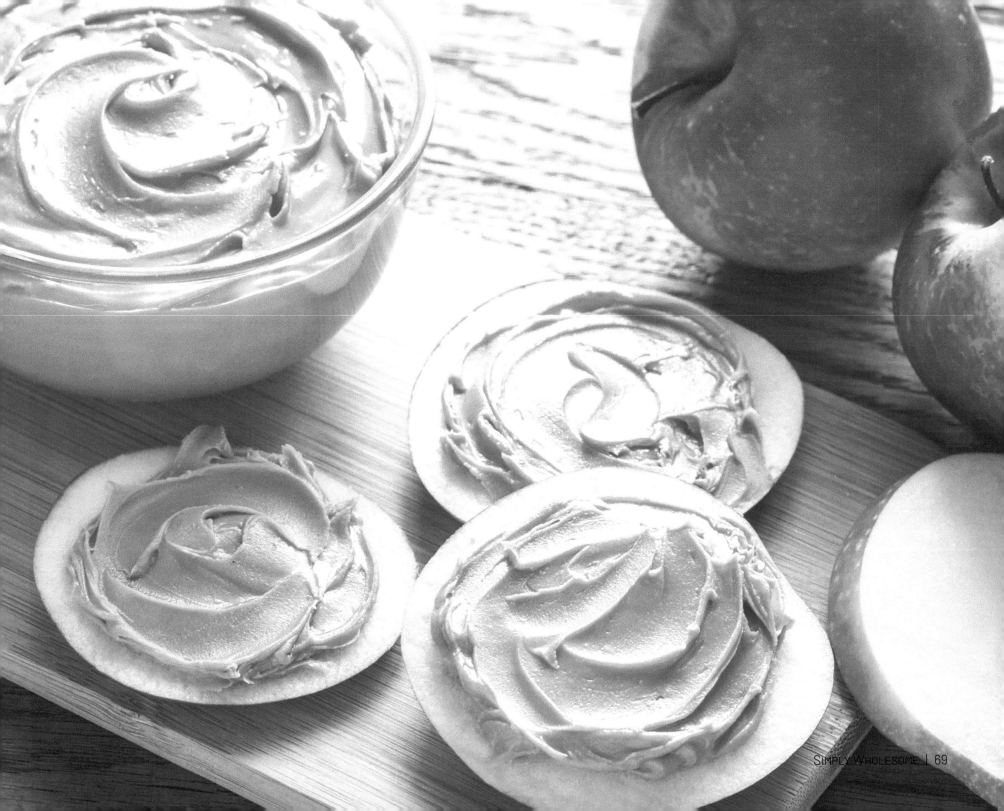

ENERGY BALLS

Feeling sluggish? About to crash? These energy balls are a perfect boost to fix that 2 p.m. slump.

Ingredients

- 1 cup medjool dates
- 1/4 cup mixed nuts
- 2 tbsp. unsweetened cocoa
- A little water

Take a drop of water and blend ingredients together in a blender until smooth.
Form mini balls and freeze.

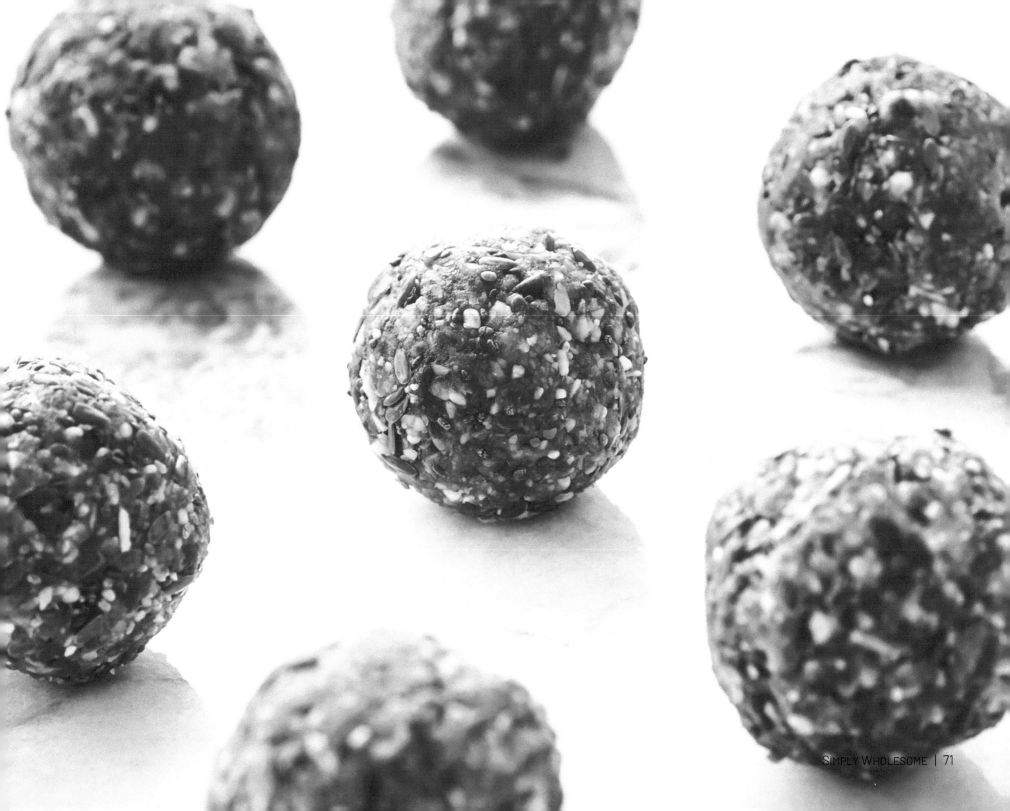

soup and side dishes for the soul

- butternut squash soup
- asparagus leek soup
- asparagus butternut squash soup
- zucchini soup
- Friday night chicken soup
- garlic roasted carrots
- zucchini chips
- cauliflower popcorn
- sweet potato & butternut squash fries
- cauliflower mash

- zucchini pizza rounds
- roasted green beans
- eat your greens
- ground turkey salad
- superpower broccoli salad
- avocado mayonnaise
- my everyday salad
- salmon avocado salad
- coleslaw

soups and
SIDE DISHES

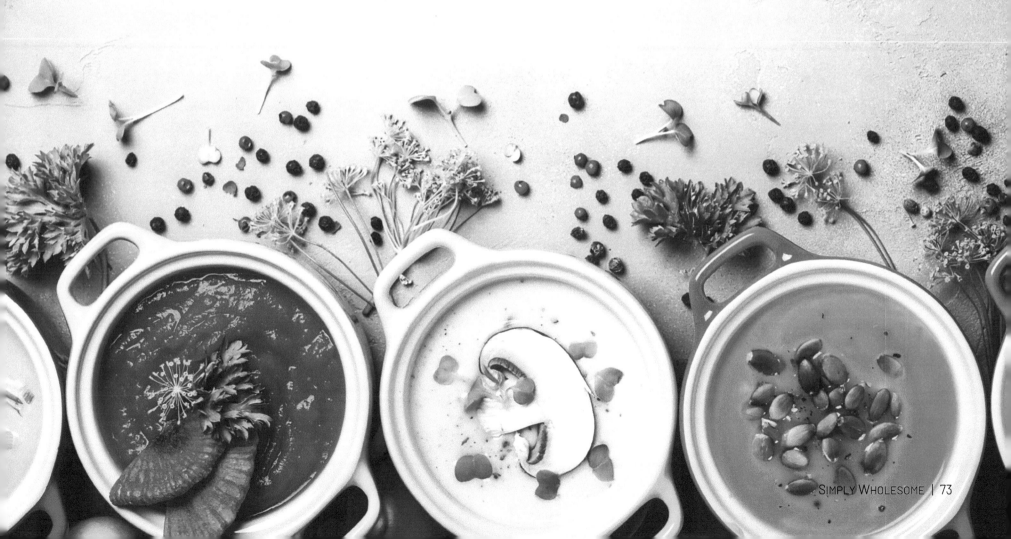

BUTTERNUT SQUASH SOUP

Remember in the beginning of this cookbook, when I told you I have a hard time getting veggies into my daily eating plan? This is how I get them in, by creating yummy soups. Now you can too!

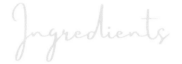

- 2 pkg. of cubed butternut squash
- 2 pkg. of cubed sweet potato
- 1 carrot
- 1 parsnip
- 1 turnip
- 1 onion
- parsley, dill, salt and pepper, to taste
- 2 cans light, unsweetened coconut milk

Add all ingredients to a soup pot. Add water to cover. Boil until soft and then blend with immersion blender. Enjoy and bon appétit!

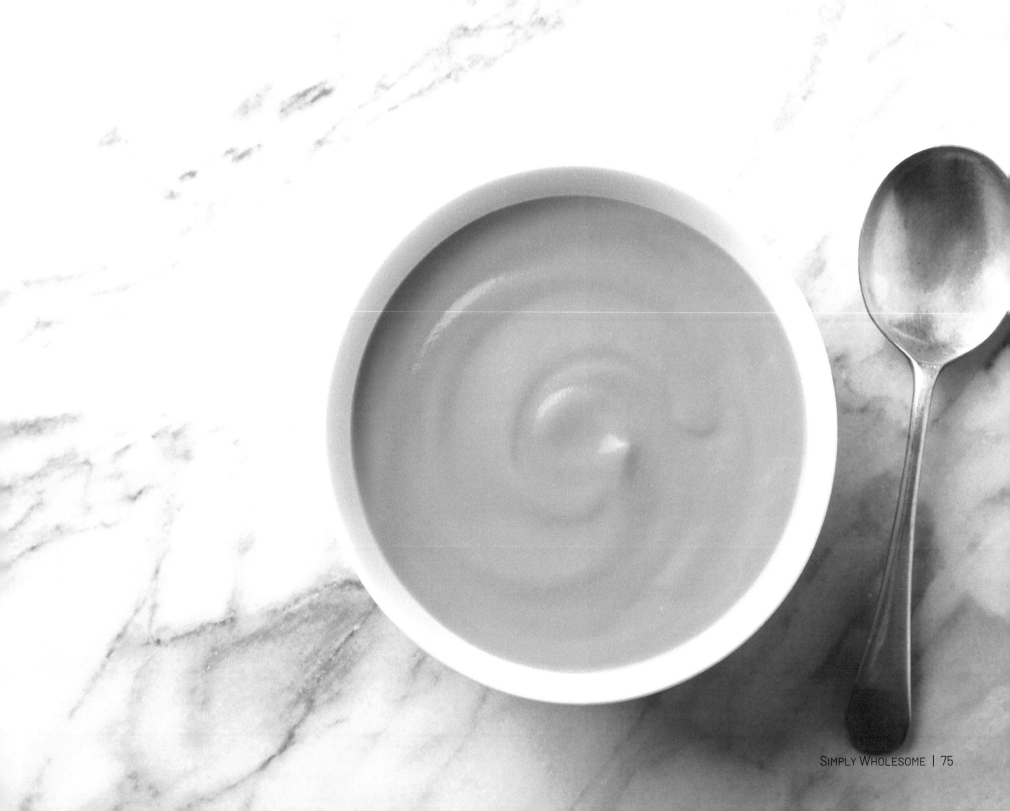

ASPARAGUS LEEK SOUP

You will see a pattern in this cookbook—I love leeks!!!

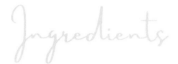

- 2 lbs. asparagus
- avocado oil spray
- 4 leeks, sliced thin
- 2 cloves garlic, minced
- 32 oz. container reduced-sodium chicken broth
- salt and pepper, to taste

Sauté leeks, stirring occasionally, until the leeks are soft, about 8 to 10 minutes.

Add garlic and cook 1 minute.

Chop the asparagus into 2-inch pieces. Add to the pot with the leeks.

Add the broth and bring to a boil.

Cover and cook about 20–25 minutes or until asparagus is very tender.

Remove from heat and puree until smooth with a blender.

Adjust salt and pepper, to taste.

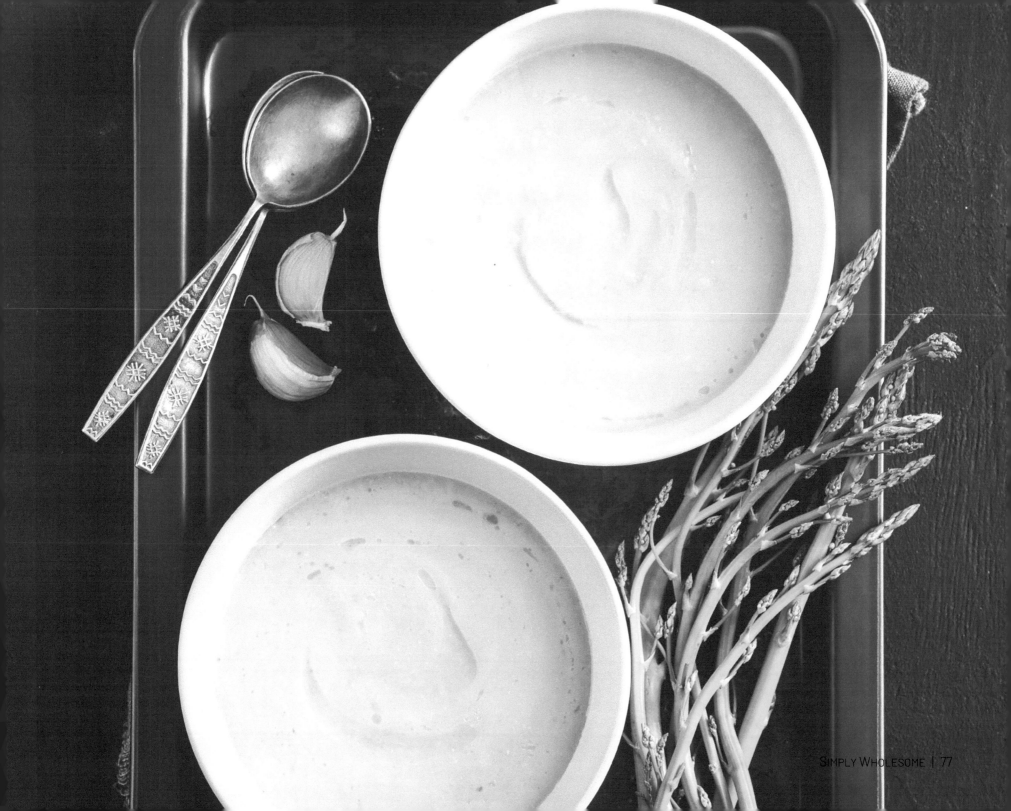

ASPARAGUS BUTTERNUT SQUASH SOUP

My client gave me this recipe and I am obsessed with it!

Ingredients

- 2 leeks, sautéed with 1 tsp. olive oil
- 3–4 stalks celery, diced
- 1 pack asparagus
- 2 packs cut-up butternut squash

Sauté the leeks, then add celery, asparagus, and squash.

Add water to cover and boil until veggies are soft.

Mash and blend with immersion blender.

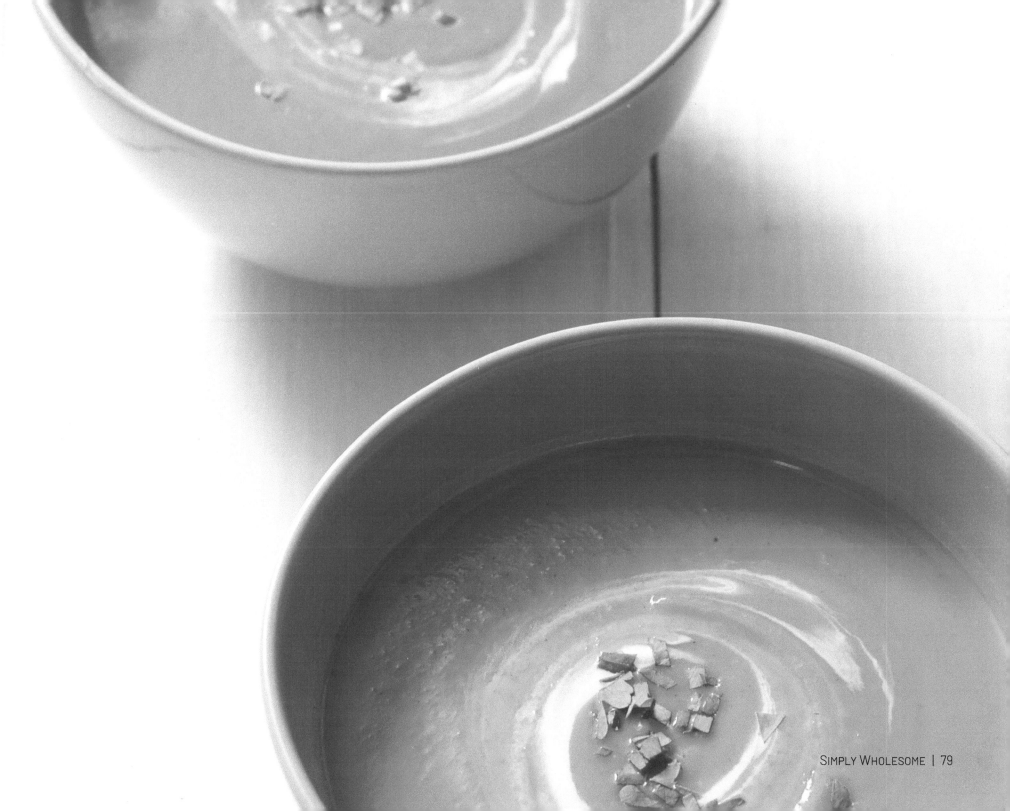

ZUCHINNI SOUP

Ingredients

- 1/2 small onion, quartered
- 2 cloves garlic
- 3 medium zucchini—skin on, cut into large chunks
- 32 oz. reduced sodium vegetable broth
- salt and pepper to taste

Combine everything in a large pot over medium heat and bring to a boil. Lower heat, cover, and simmer until tender, about 20 minutes.

Remove from heat and puree with immersion blender until smooth.

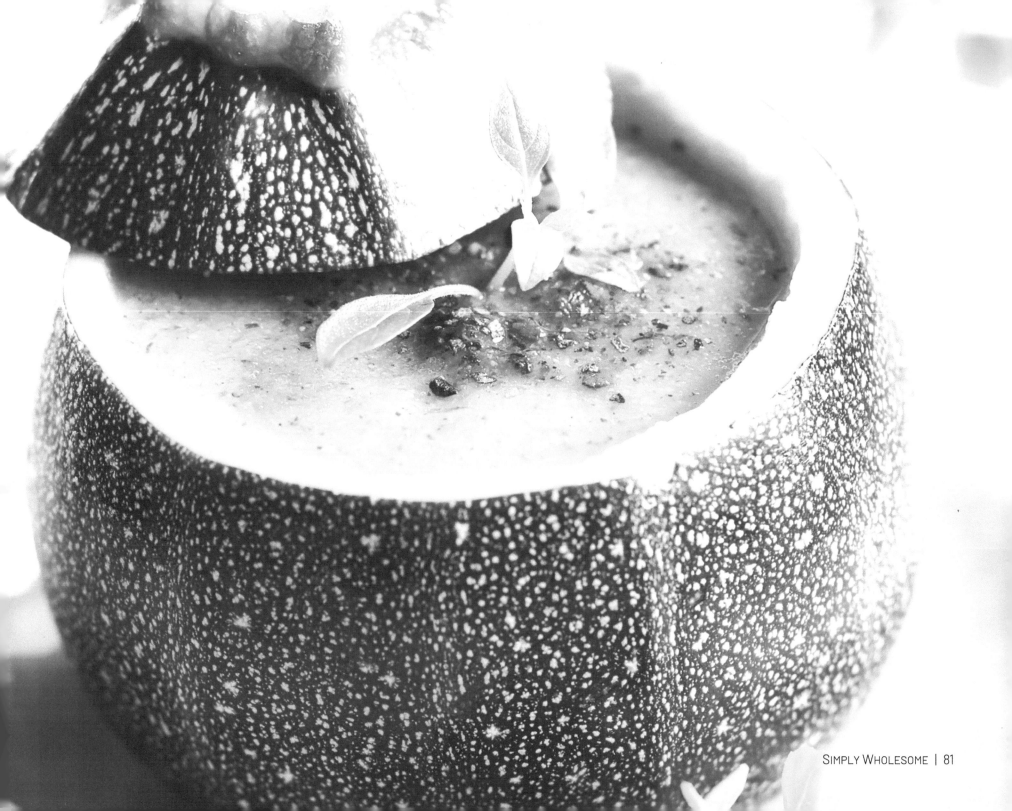

FRIDAY NIGHT CHICKEN SOUP

This chicken soup is a winner for two reasons: 1. My whole family loves it—that never happens; and 2. It's got healthy protein, healthy carbs; and healthy fat, all in one—chicken cutlet (protein), barley (carbohydrate), and olive oil (fat). Plus, it is so filling, you won't need to eat anything else. We pretty much have this soup every week.

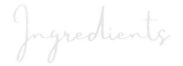

Ingredients

- 1 large onion, diced
- 1 tbsp. olive oil
- 3 stalks celery, diced
- 1 1/2 tsp. minced garlic, fresh
- 3 medium carrots, diced
- 3 medium zucchini diced, skin on
- 10 cups water
- 1 cup barley, rinsed
- 1 lb. chicken cutlets
- 1 tbsp. kosher salt
- 1 tbsp. parsley flakes, dried
- 1 tsp. onion powder
- 1/2 tsp. cumin
- 1/2 tsp. paprika
- 1/2 tsp. pepper

Sauté the onion, celery, and garlic with the olive oil spray for 3 minutes.

Add the vegetables, barley, and chicken cutlets (leave them whole) with all the spices. Combine.

Add water. Bring to a boil for an hour, until chicken is cooked and vegetables are soft.

Remove the chicken from the soup and shred it with a fork. The chicken should be very soft and easy to shred.

Put it back in the soup and serve hot.

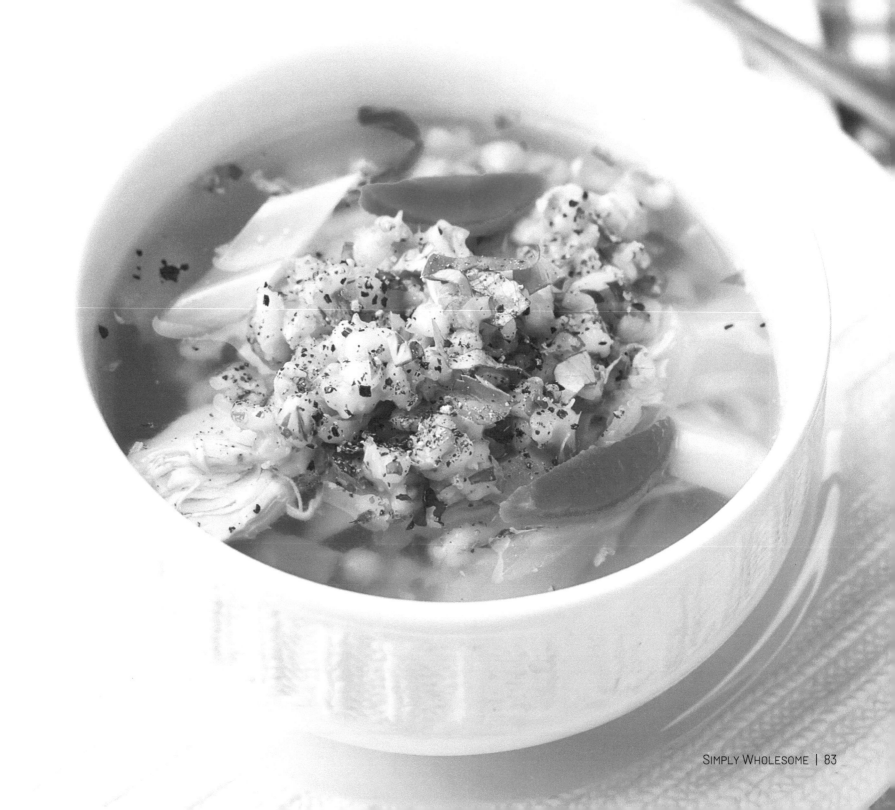

GARLIC ROASTED CARROTS

Ingredients

- 2 bags orange carrots (or tri-colored)
- 2 tbsp. olive oil
- 2 tbsp. light balsamic vinegar
- 5 cloves garlic, minced
- 1 tsp. dried thyme
- Kosher salt and freshly ground black pepper, to taste
- 2 tbsp. chopped parsley leaves

Spread spice mixture onto carrots.

Roast on baking sheet at 425 °F for 30–40 minutes.

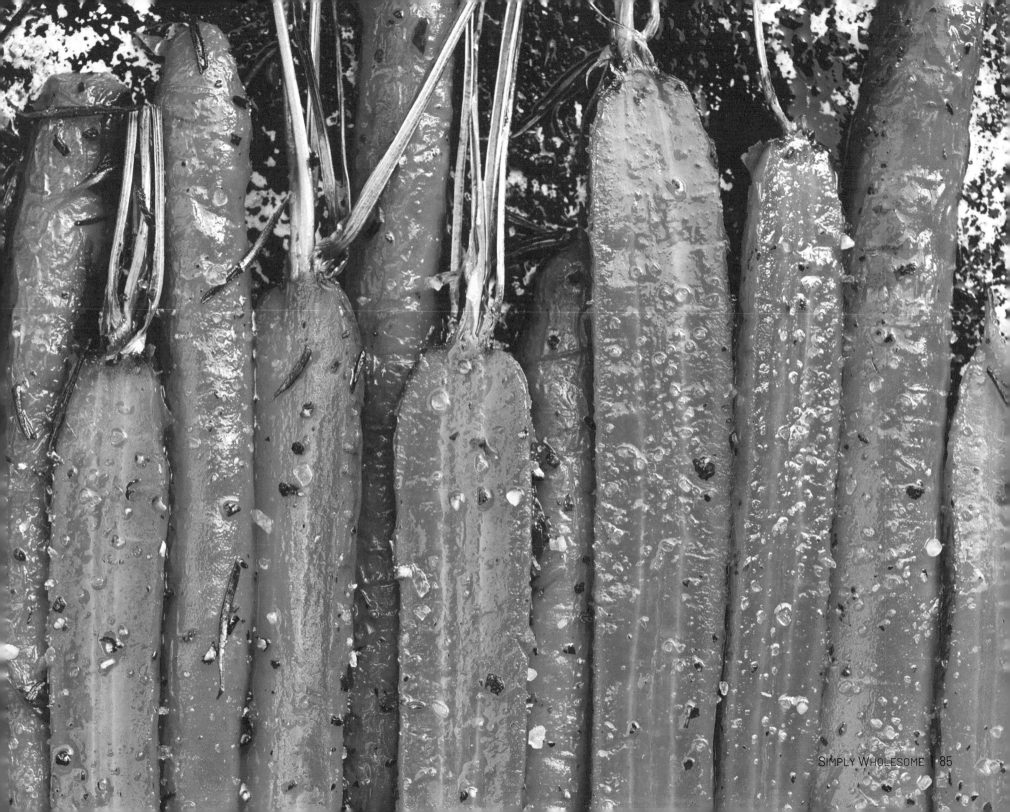

ZUCHINNI CHIPS

- 1–2 large zucchini, sliced thin
- Olive oil spray
- Trader Joe's Everything but The Bagel spice

Sprinkle all over and bake at 350 °F until crispy.

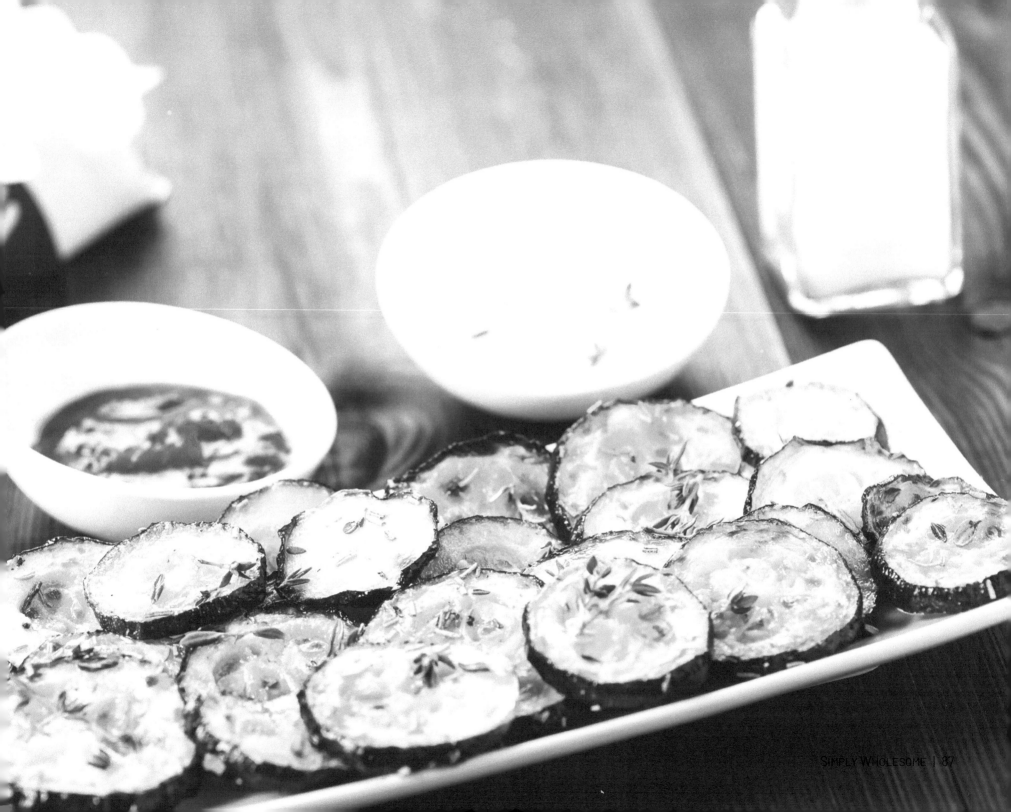

CAULIFLOWER POPCORN

I love posting recipes with superpower ingredients, like this one:
Turmeric has powerful anti-inflammatory effects and is a strong antioxidant.

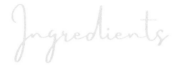

- 1 tsp. sea salt
- 2 tsp. sugar
- 1/4–1/2 tsp. ground turmeric
- 1/2 tsp. paprika
- 1/4 tsp. onion powder
- 1/4 tsp. garlic powder
- 1–2 tbsp. light olive oil
- 1 bag frozen cauliflower

Preheat oven to 450 °F. Line a pan with parchment paper.

In a large bowl combine salt, sugar, turmeric, paprika, onion, garlic powder, and oil.

Place in a single layer on a baking sheet.

Roast uncovered, 30–35 minutes.

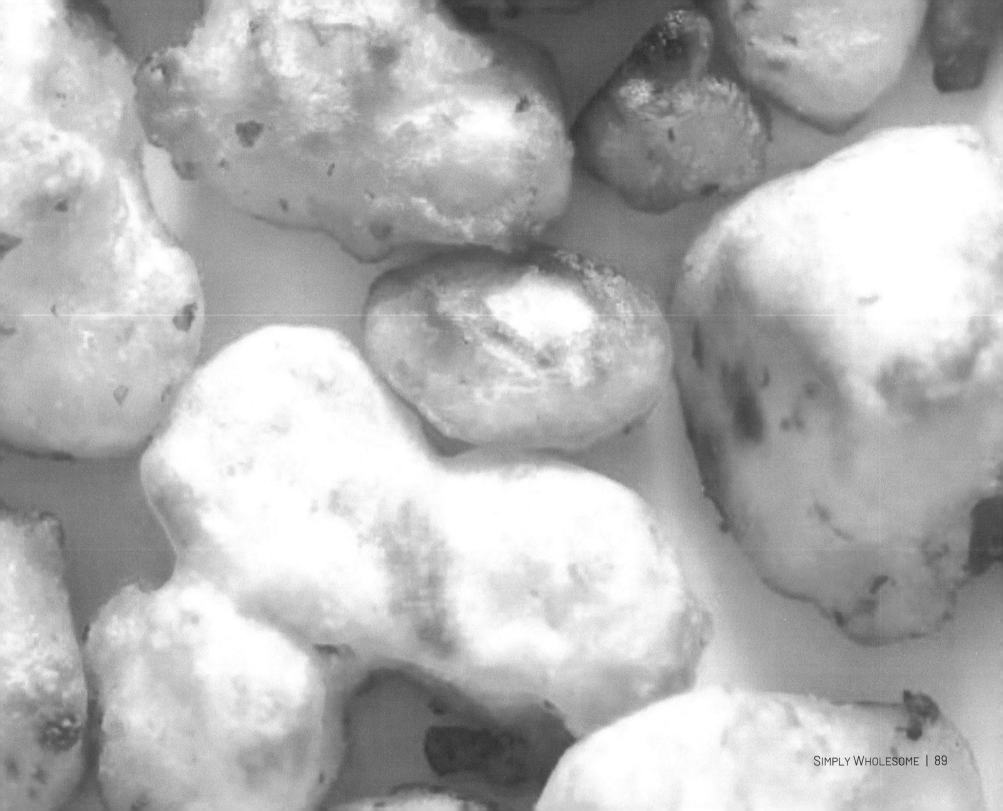

SWEET POTATO AND BUTTERNUT SQUASH FRIES

Before I discovered this recipe, I never ate sweet potato. Knowing that sweet potato is one of the healthiest foods out there, I needed to find a way to eat them. These barely make it to the table. As soon as they come out of the oven, it's a mad dash for everyone.

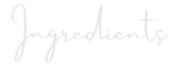

Ingredients

- Sweet potato and butternut squash, sliced into strips (some stores have it already precut! Get those and save your fingers!)
- Kosher salt—sprinkle around
- Thyme—sprinkle around
- Olive oil—maybe a tsp;—smear all over
- Spread the fries evenly on a baking sheet, so they don't overlap
- Bake at 425 °F around 45 minutes

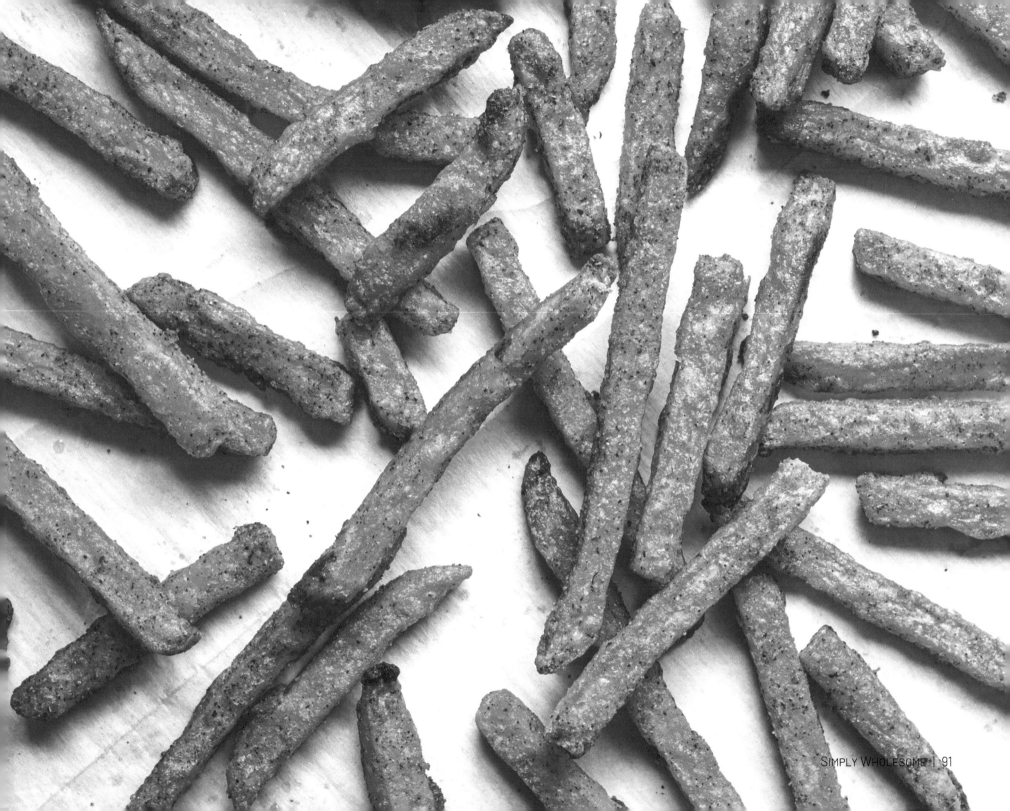

CAULIFLOWER MASH

Kind of like mashed potatoes, but with fewer carbs and more nutrients.

Ingredients

- 1 bag frozen cauliflower
- salt and pepper, for sprinkling
- Olive oil—drizzle or use the spray
- 6 garlic cloves

Preheat oven to 350 °F. Throw all ingredients into a 9 x 13 pan.

Cover and bake for 1 1/2 hours or until cauliflower is super soft.

Mash with a fork and indulge.

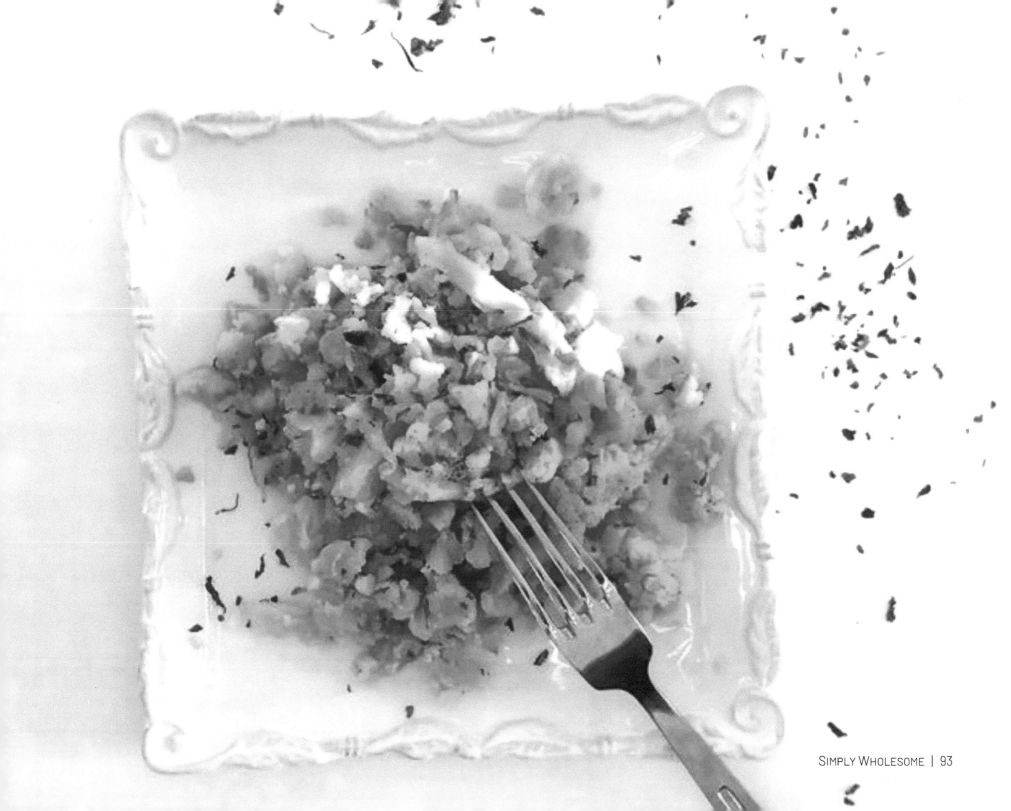

ZUCHINNI PIZZA ROUNDS

Ingredients

- 1–2 zucchini, sliced into rounds
- marinara sauce
- reduced fat mozzarella cheese
- salt and pepper
- avocado oil spray
- pizza spice

Arrange zucchini slices in a single layer on a prepared baking sheet.

Spray with avocado oil spray and sprinkle with salt and pepper.

Bake at 450 °F until just crisp-tender, about 5 minutes.

Top each slice with marinara sauce, cheese, and pizza spice.

Bake at 450 °F for about 8–10 minutes, until cheese is melted and zucchini is soft.

Broil for 1–2 minutes to brown cheese. Serve immediately!

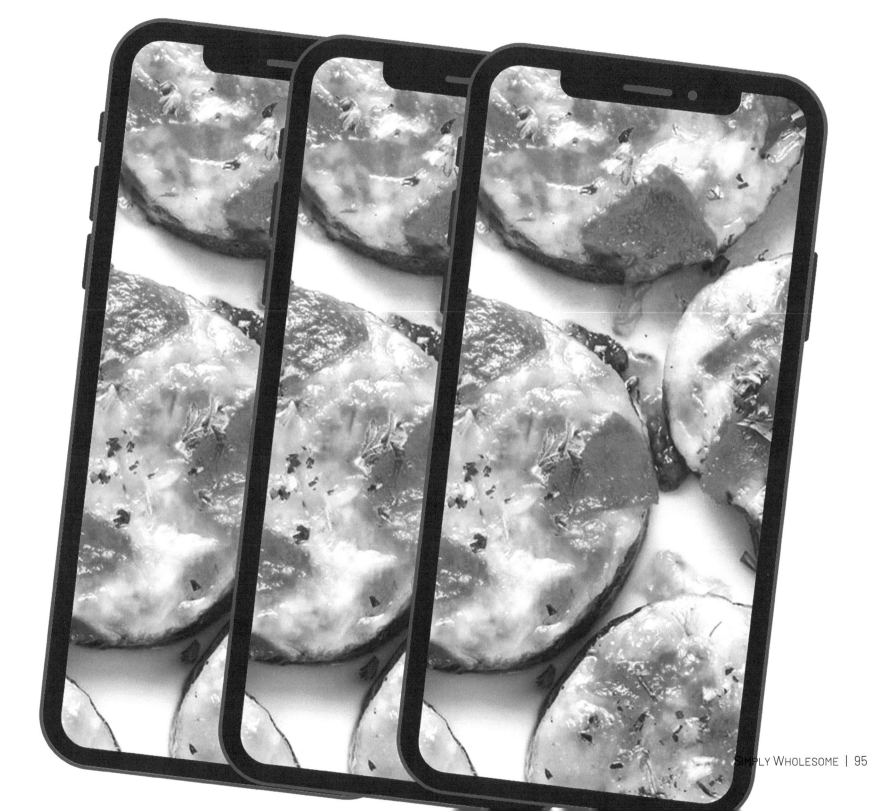

ROASTED GREEN BEANS

Another weekly staple in my house. These also barely make it to the table. I find that I always need to make another batch, because I keep going back for just one more.

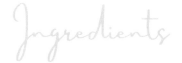

Ingredients

- 1 package of green beans
- Trader Joe's Everything but The Bagel spice
- Nutritional yeast
- Onion powder
- Olive oil/avocado oil spray

Arrange green beans on a flat baking pan.

Spray green beans with oil. Sprinkle spices and nutritional yeast. Smear the green beans until everything is coated. Bake in oven at 550 °F for 20–25 minutes. Check them regularly. The green beans should be crispy, but not burnt.

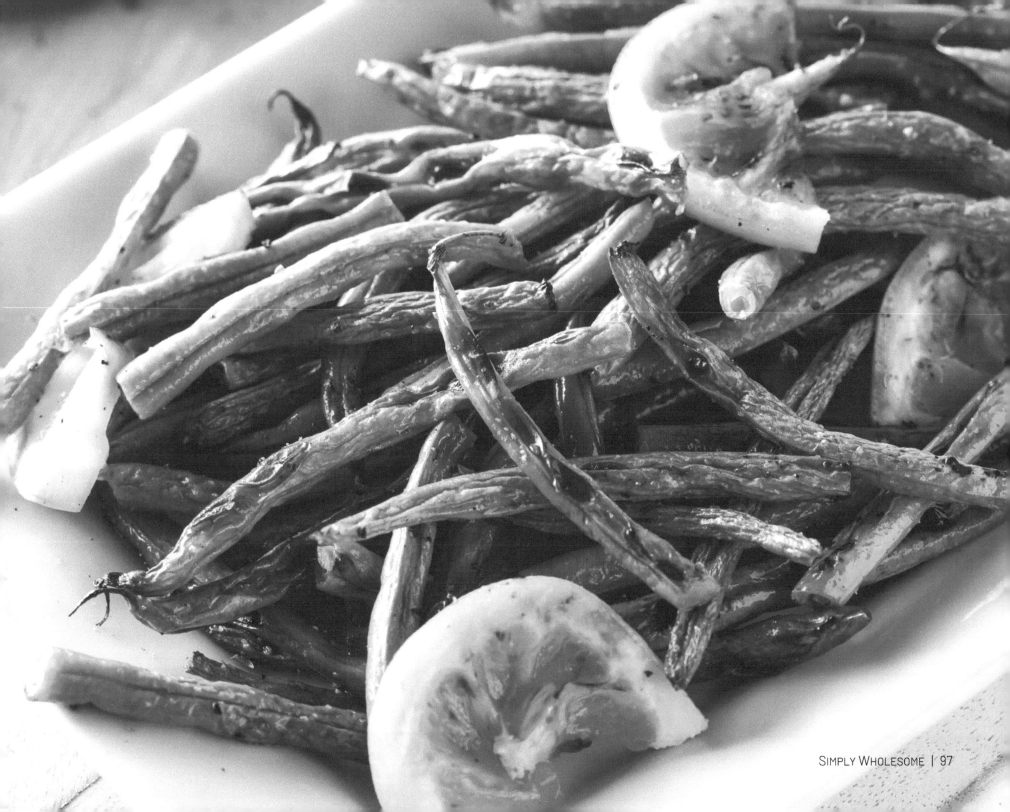

EAT YOUR GREENS

- 1 bag mixed greens
- 4 radishes, thinly sliced
- 1 avocado, thinly sliced
- 1 large cucumber, thinly sliced
- 1 bunch chives, minced
- 1 tbsp. pomegranate seeds

Dressing:
- 1/3 cup light olive oil
- 2 tbsp. Dijon mustard
- 2 tbsp. lemon juice
- 2 tsp. honey
- 1 scallion, minced
- 1/4 tsp. salt

In a small bowl, whisk together ingredients for the dressing, set aside.

Arrange mixed greens in bowl. Top with radishes, cucumber, avocado, chives and sprinkle with pomegranate seeds.

Drizzle with dressing right before serving and enjoy!

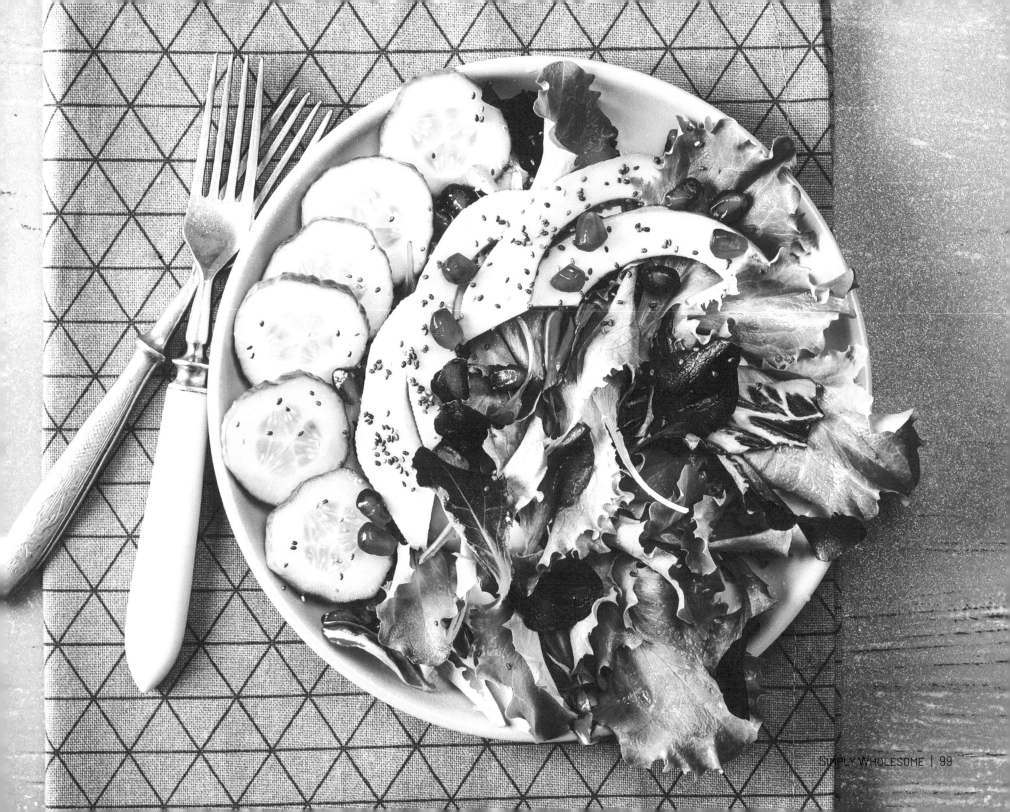

GROUND TURKEY SALAD

1 lb. ground lean turkey:

Season with paprika, garlic powder, salt, ketchup, Trader Joe's Everything but The Bagel spice, and onion powder and add 1 egg. (Just sprinkle the spices around, no exact measurements needed).

Place 1 tbsp. olive oil into the pan and brown the meat.

Add 1/4 cup tomato basil marinara sauce into pan and mix.

Salad (add as much as what you prefer):

- Mixed greens
- Cherry tomatoes, Scallions
- Terra chips or beet chips
- Feel free to add avocado, red onion, or whatever else you want.

Dressing:

- 1 tbsp. honey mustard light from Saladmate

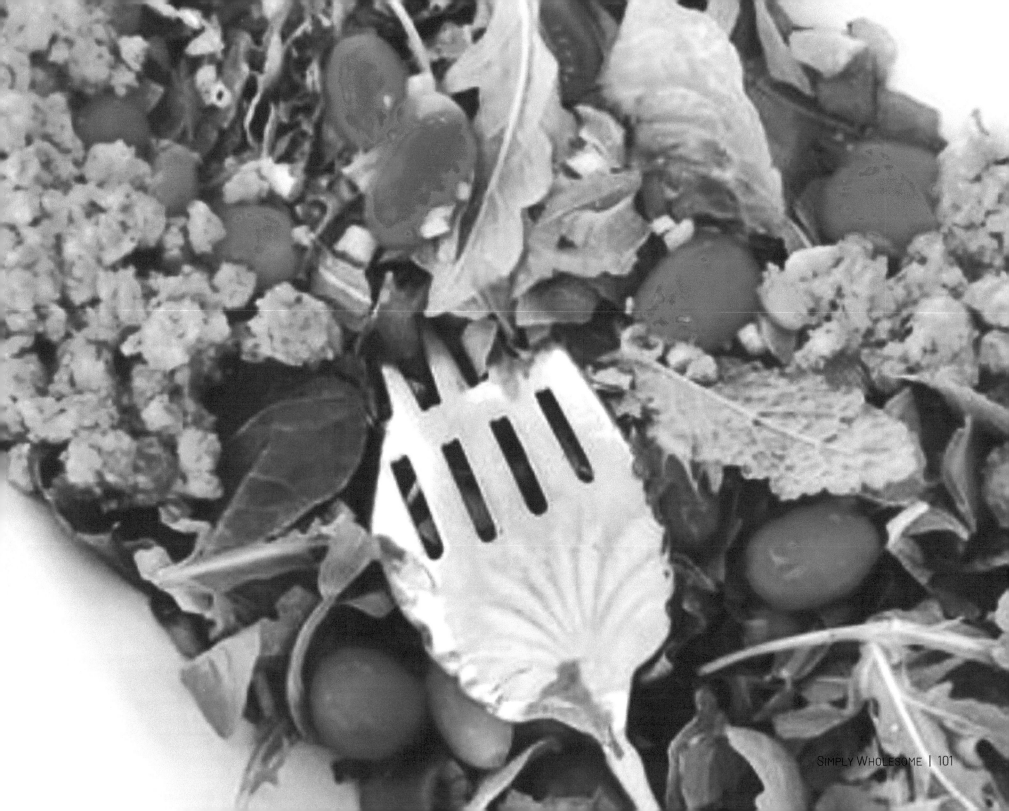

SUPERPOWER BROCCOLI SALAD

Another super power ingredient in here: cumin. Cumin is a good source of Vitamin A, calcium, and iron.
It also aids with digestion, and cholesterol control and has many more benefits.

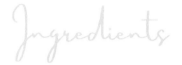

- 1/4 cup thinly sliced red onion
- 1/2 tsp. ground cumin
- 1/3 cup light mayonnaise
- 2 tbsp. tahini
- 2 tbsp. light olive oil
- 1 tbsp. lemon juice
- 1/2 tsp. salt
- 1/2 tsp. ground pepper
- 8 oz. broccoli florets
- 1 (15 oz.) low sodium chickpeas, rinsed
- 1/2 cup pomegranate seeds

Toast cumin in pan over medium heat for 1–2 minutes. Transfer cumin into large bowl.

Mix mayonnaise, tahini, oil, lemon juice, and salt and pepper in a separate bowl. Whisk until smooth.

Add broccoli, chickpeas, red onion, and pomegranate seeds to the cumin. Add dressing on top. Toss to combine.

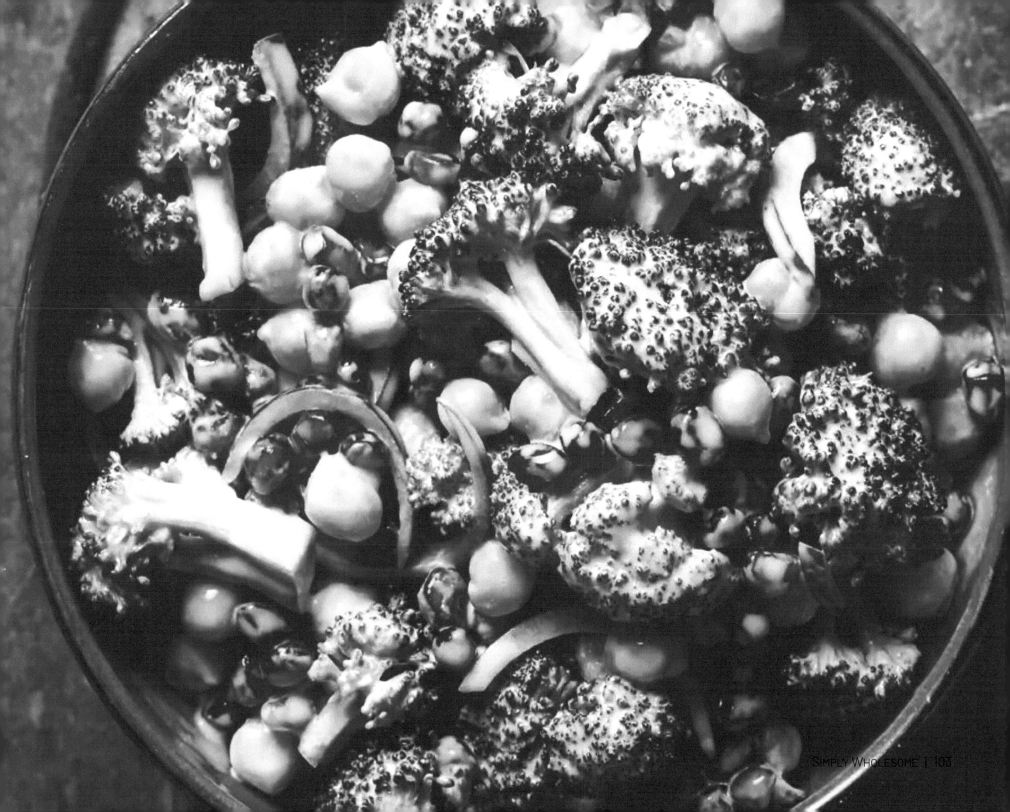

AVOCADO MAYONNAISE

Ingredients

- 1 ripe avocado, peeled
- 3 tbsp. lemon juice
- 2 tsp. Dijon mustard
- 1/2 tsp. sea salt
- 1/3 cup olive oil

Blend avocados, lemon juice, salt, and mustard until smooth. Slowly add in the olive oil and continue blending.

Feel free to use this on whatever you use mayonnaise for (bread, salads, tuna, etc.)

Store in an airtight container in the fridge.

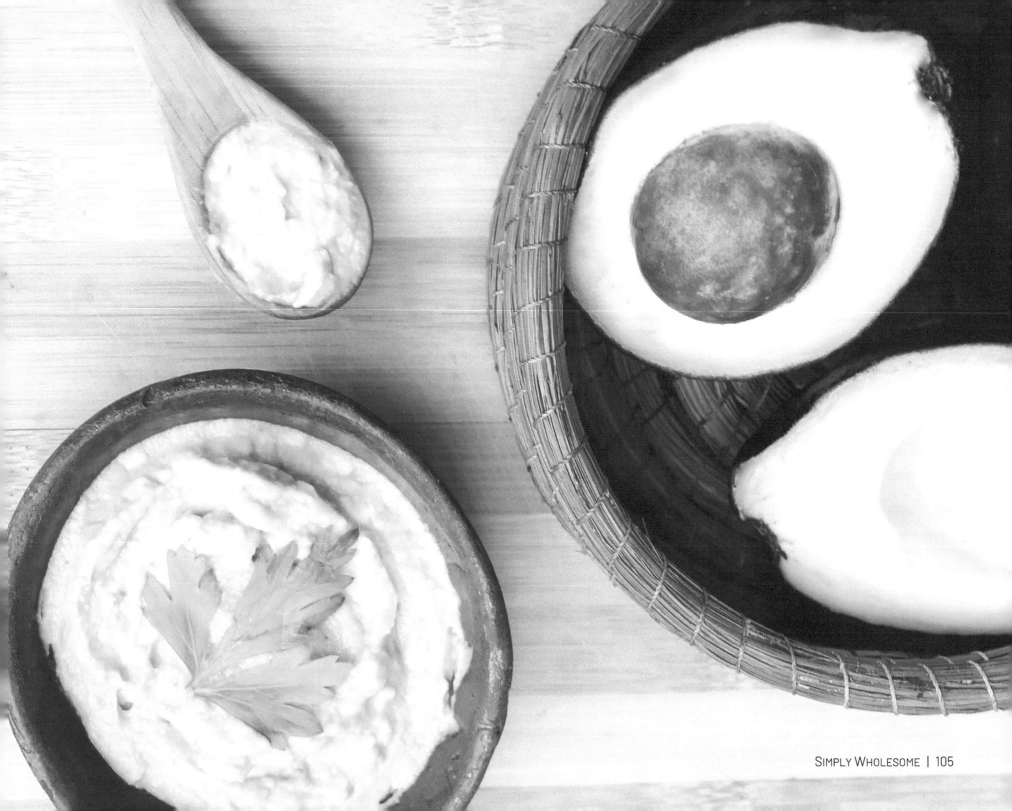

MY EVERYDAY SALAD

I am not kidding when I say I have this salad every day. I hardly ever get bored of it. I personally don't like feta.
See, I told you I'm picky. But I added it in for you guys as an extra protein boost.
Sometimes I'll switch it up by taking out one of the ingredients, but basically this is my go-to salad.

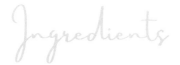

- Mixed greens
- A handful of purple cabbage, shredded
- 1 scallion, diced
- 5 medium strawberries or nectarines, depending on the season
- 1 tbsp. walnuts or sliced almonds
- A handful crushed beet chips or Terra chips
- 1/4 cup feta (optional)
- 1 tbsp. sunflower seeds or pumpkin seeds
- 1 tbsp. light honey mustard dressing, Saladmate brand

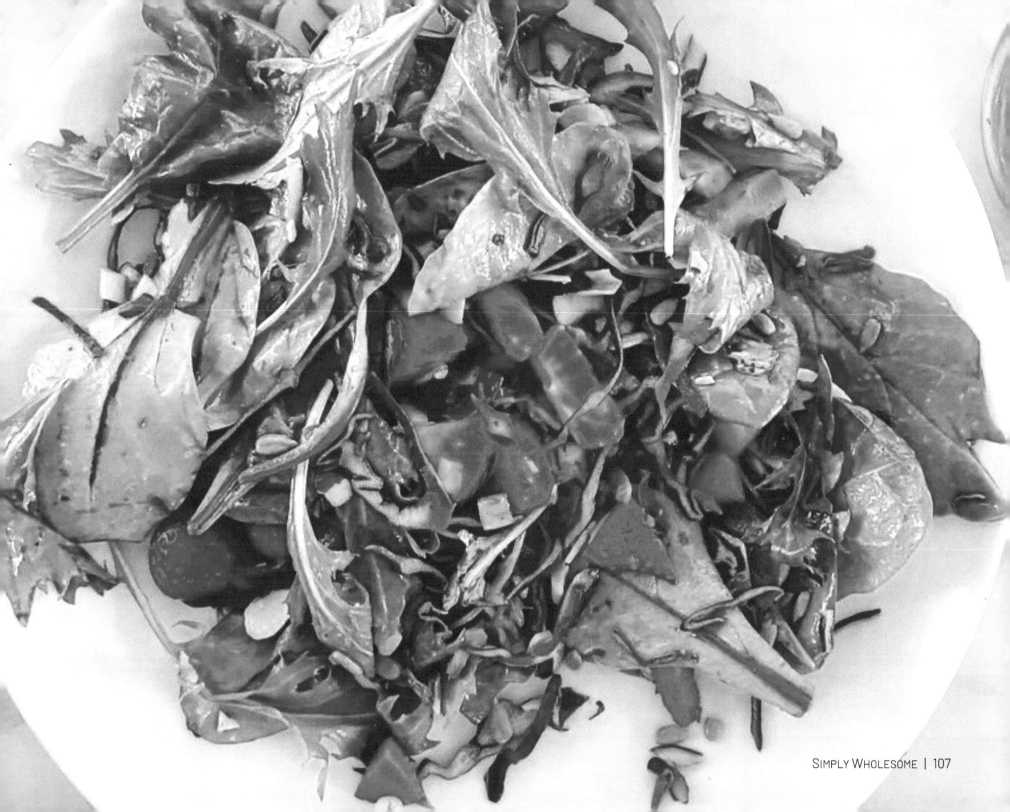

SALMON AVOCADO SALAD

I love making salads that look pretty and taste yummy.
I mean look at the colors here, the green, the purple, and the red from the tomatoes and pomegranate seeds.
This salad is Instagram worthy!

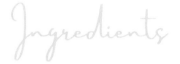

- 4 salmon fillets
- 1 tbsp. honey mustard, split
- 3/4 tsp. dried parsley
- 1/2 tsp. kosher salt and black pepper
- 1/4 cup red onion, chopped
- 2 tsp. light olive oil
- 2 tbsp. apple cider vinegar
- 1/8 tsp. garlic powder
- 1 cup cherry tomatoes
- 1 avocado
- Mixed greens
- 1/2 cup shredded red cabbage
- pomegranate seeds, (optional)

Season salmon with 2 tsp. honey mustard, 1/2 tsp. parsley, and 1/4 tsp. salt and pepper.

Broil salmon 6–7 minutes.

Combine red onion with olive oil, 1 1/2 tbsp. vinegar, 1 tsp. remaining honey mustard, 1/4 tsp. parsley, and 1/4 tsp. salt and pepper. Let sit 5 minutes.

Pour over mixed greens, tomato, avocado slices, cabbage, and pomegranate seeds. Dig in!

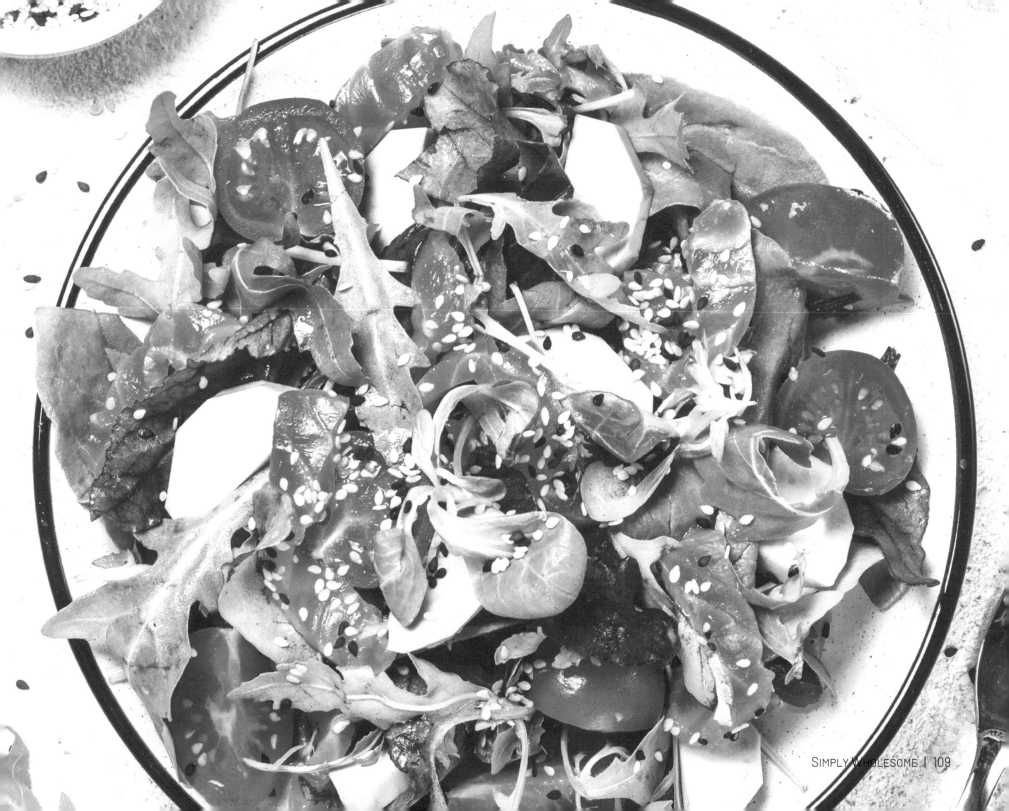

COLESLAW

Perfect for Rosh Hashanah, with all its simanim

Ingredients

- 1 bag of coleslaw
- 1 scallion, diced
- 1 green apple, sliced thin or julienned
- 1 tbsp. sliced almonds
- 1/4 cup pomegranate seeds
- 1–2 tbsp. light honey mustard dressing

- grilled chicken

- pistachio—crusted salmon

- air—fried chicken tenders

- salmon with leeks

- healthy pizza

- 3-ingredient salmon

- Chinese chicken

- pargiyot

- tilapia

- best grilled chicken

- broccoli cutlets

- melt-in your-mouth grilled chicken

- oven—roasted salmon

- turkey meatballs

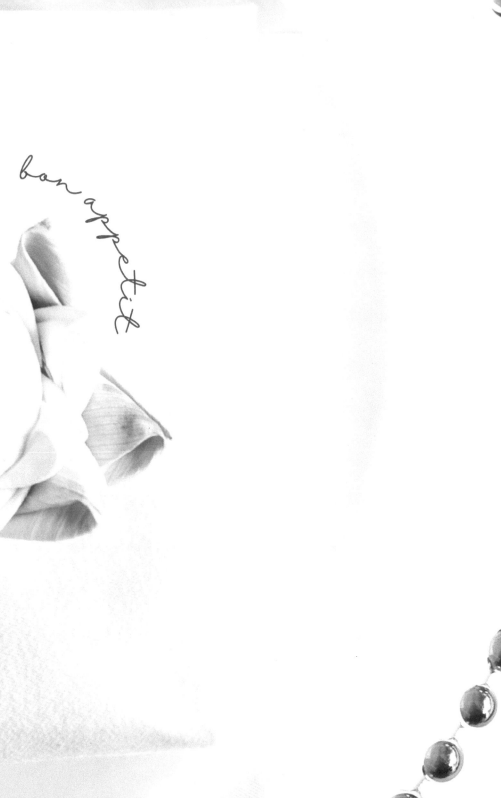

bon appetit

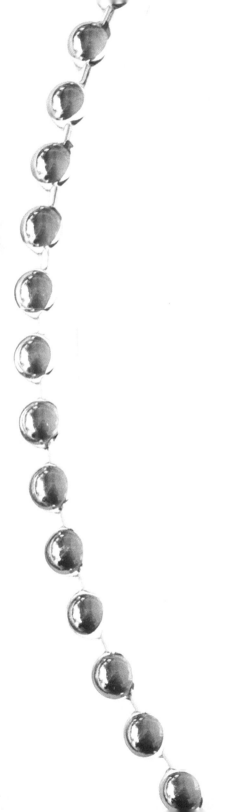

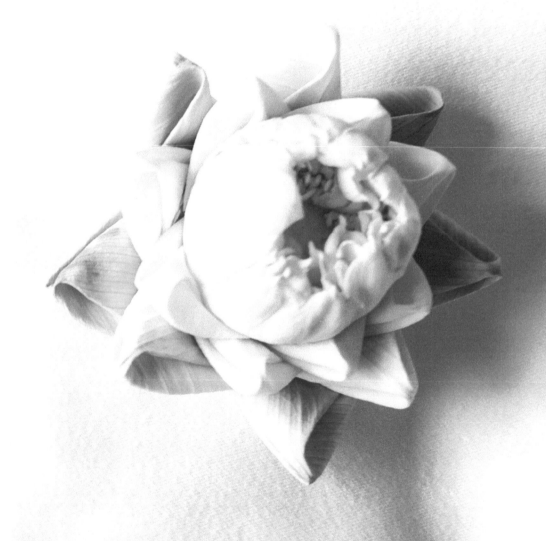

What's for dinner?

GRILLED CHICKEN

These are amazing. They come out so soft and juicy. Just make sure you do not overcook them.

Ingredients

- Boneless chicken breasts (get the ones that are sliced thin from the butcher)
- 1/2 tsp. paprika
- 1 tbsp. dried parsley
- 1 tbsp. sesame seeds
- 2 tbsp. bread crumbs (I used panko)
- 2 tbsp. crushed garlic
- 2 tbsp. olive oil
- 1 1/2 tsp. minced onion
- 1/2 tsp. kosher salt

Mix all ingredients in a bowl. Place coated chicken breast on baking sheet.
Bake at 425 °F for 15 minutes.

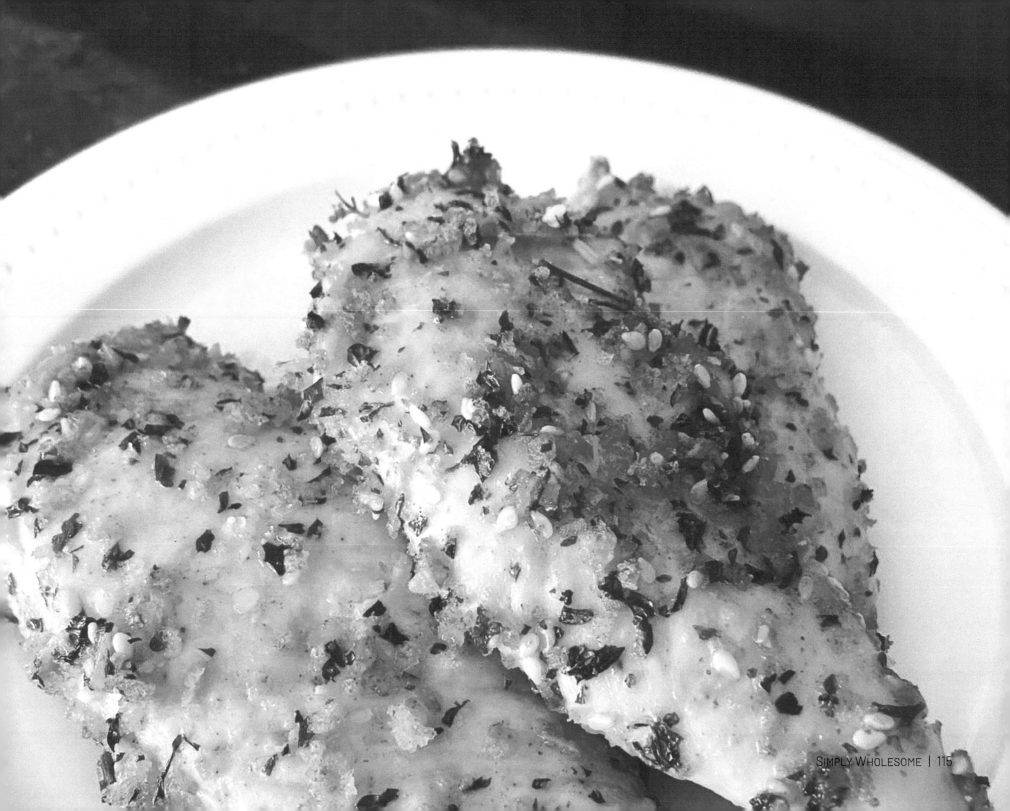

PISTACHIO-CRUSTED SALMON

Are you a full time working mom? These can be made in an air fryer! You can make the sauce first, then marinate the salmon and as soon as you get home, pop it in the air fryer and supper is ready!

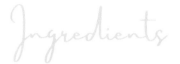

Ingredients

- 4 salmon filets
- 1 tbsp. honey
- 1 tbsp. Dijon mustard
- 2–3 cloves minced garlic
- 1/4 cup panko
- 1/2 cup crushed pistachios
- Salt, pepper, garlic powder, onion powder, and paprika (I just eyeball these)
- Lemon slices, optional

Pat salmon dry. Mix honey, garlic, and mustard together and rub on salmon.

Add panko, pistachios, and seasonings to a bowl and mix.

Coat salmon in the pistachio mix; then place into an air fryer and top off with lemon slices. Fry at 390 °F, no preheat, for about 7–9 minutes (depending on thickness).

Cover with tin foil halfway through if it starts to brown and enjoy!

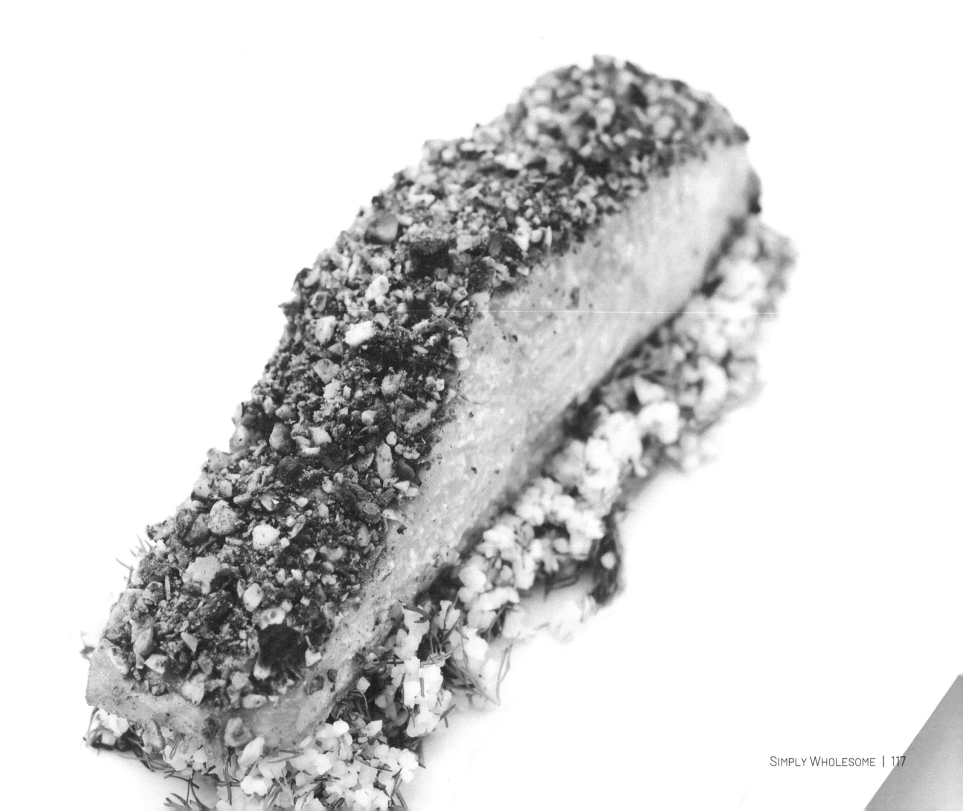

AIR-FRIED CHICKEN TENDERS

Can fried chicken cutlets be healthy? Yup, now they can.

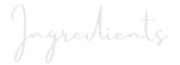

Ingredients

- 12 chicken cutlets
- 2 large eggs, beaten
- 1 tsp. kosher salt
- black pepper, to taste
- 1/2 cup seasoned panko crumbs

Season chicken with salt and pepper.

Place eggs in a bowl. In a second bowl, pour the panko crumbs in.

Dip chicken in the egg, then into the panko crumbs.

Shake off any excess and place on a large dish or cutting board.

Preheat air fryer to 400 °F.

In batches, cook the chicken 5–6 minutes per side, until the chicken is cooked through and golden on the outside.

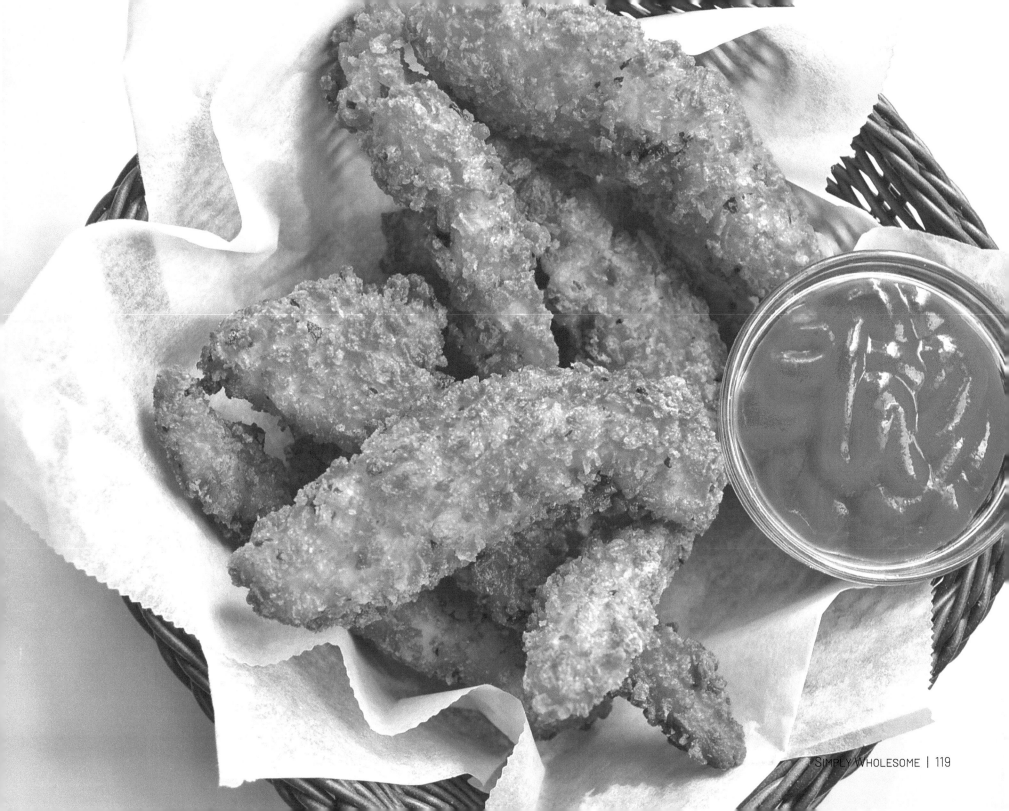

SALMON WITH LEEKS

Best recipe—hands down!

Ingredients

- 4 salmon fillets, no skin
- 1 tbsp. coconut or avocado oil
- salt and pepper
- 3 leeks, sliced into half rings
- honey

Heat up the avocado/coconut oil in a pan. Sauté the leeks until light brown and soft.

Sprinkle salt and pepper over fillets. Drizzle honey over salmon.

Spread sautéed leeks over salmon.

Bake uncovered at 400 °F for 25 minutes.

This dish can be served warm or cold.

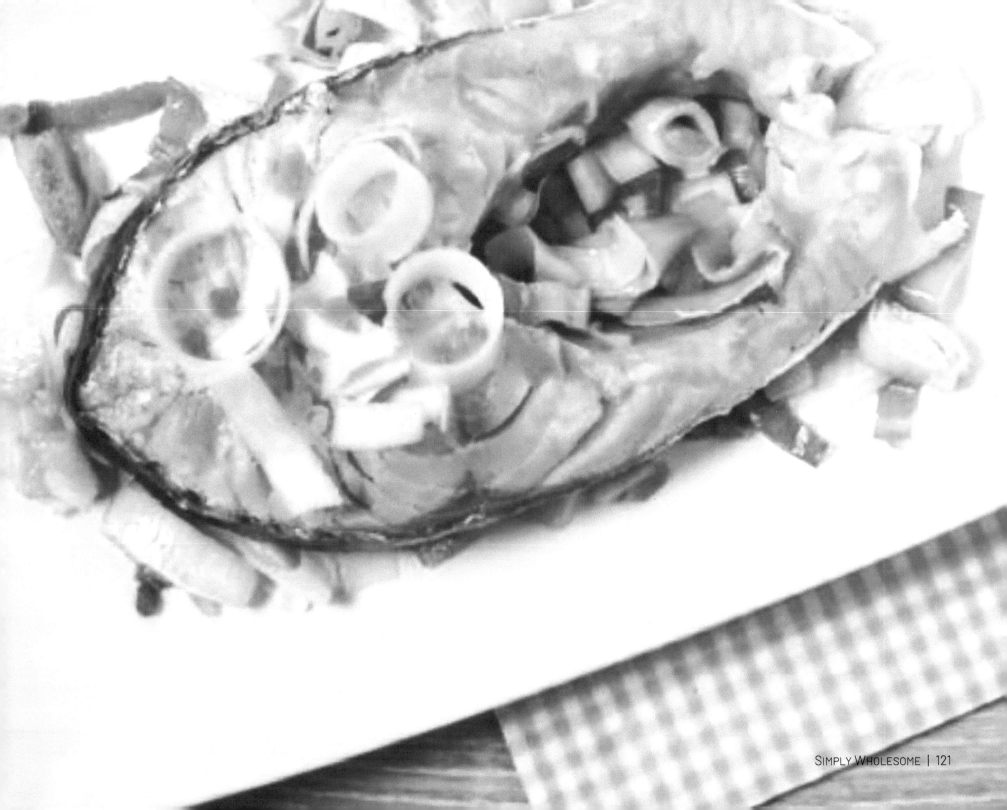

HEALTHY PIZZA

Yes, I'll have a slice or two...

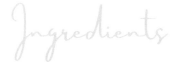

- 1 whole-wheat wrap (I use @nutritionbytanya)
- 1 tbsp. fat-free pizza sauce
- 1/4 cup reduced fat mozzarella shredded cheese
- pizza spice

Spread pizza sauce on wrap.

Sprinkle shredded cheese on top.

Sprinkle pizza spice as to your liking.

Put in toaster oven, heat at 450 °F for less than 5 minutes, and garnish with some greens!

3-INGREDIENT SALMON

Another pattern in this cookbook: most of my recipes have very few ingredients, making preparation a breeze.

Ingredients

- 4 salmon fillets
- 2 tbsp. Smart Balance butter
- Trader Joe's Everything but The Bagel spice
- Light mayonnaise

Add 1 tbsp. of mayonnaise around all the fillets. Sprinkle the spice and smear each fillet until coated.

Add the butter to the pan and wait until it melts.

Add each fillet of salmon to the pan and cook until it is no longer raw. It should be a light pink.

This can be served at room temperature or straight out of the pan—like I do!

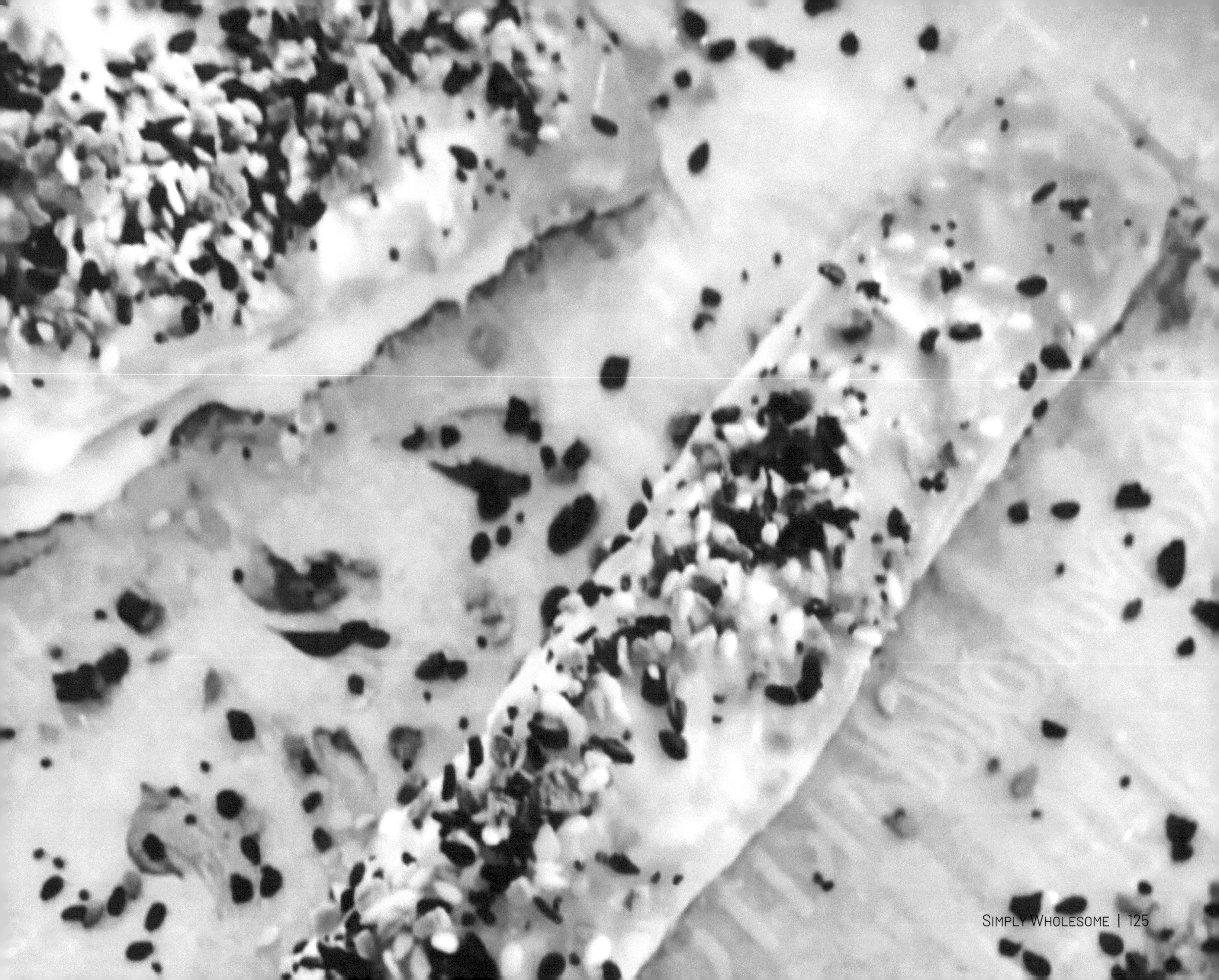

CHINESE CHICKEN

No need to order in, pick up your chopsticks and dig in. So good, and the best part: it takes 5 minutes to make!

Ingredients

- 2 packages cut-up chicken cutlets,
- 4 scallions, diced
- 1 tbsp. minced fresh garlic
- 1 tsp. crushed red pepper flakes

Sauce:
- 1 1/2 cups chicken broth, low sodium (I use Imagine brand)
- 4 tbsp. cornstarch
- 4 tbsp. stevia/truvia
- 2 tbsp. red wine vinegar
- 4 tbsp. coconut aminos
- 1 tsp. ginger

Sauté scallions, garlic, and red pepper flakes in a large frying pan.

Add in chicken and continue to sauté until chicken isn't pink anymore.

Meanwhile, prepare the sauce. Add sauce to chicken and let it boil. Do not mix the chicken until sauce starts to thicken. Mix the chicken with the sauce. It should be fully coated.

Note: red pepper flakes are very spicy, you may need to play around with the amount the first couple of times you make this dish.

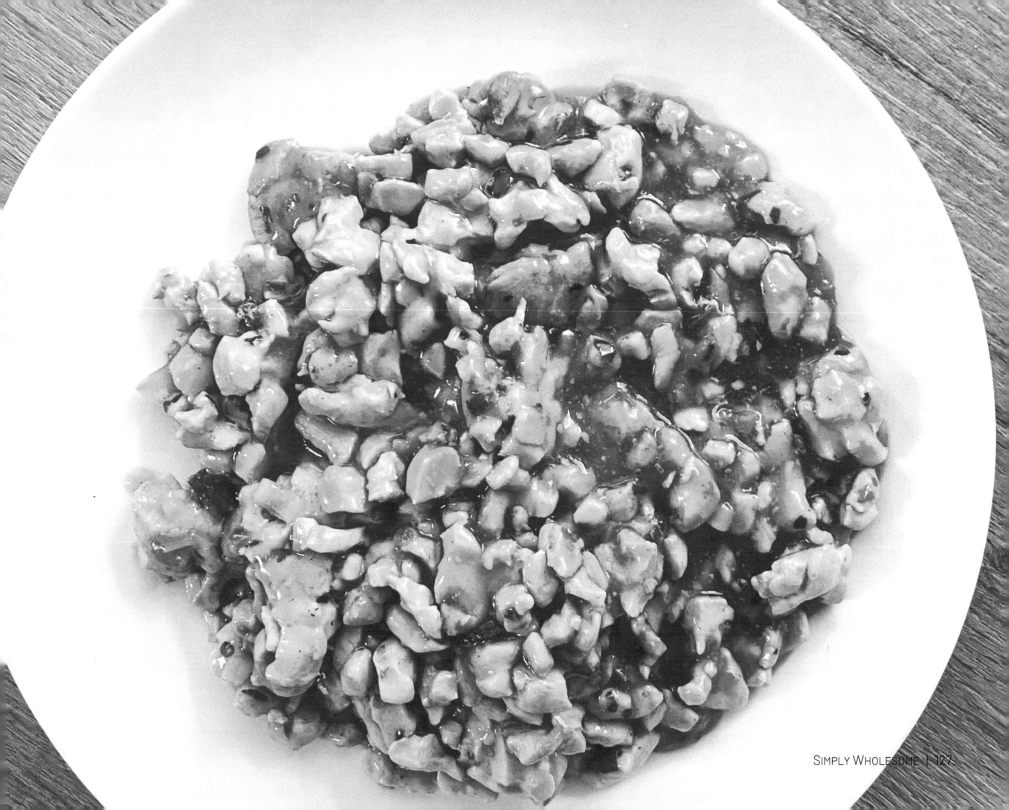

HONEY MUSTARD GRILLED PARGIYOT

- 3 pounds chicken pargiyot

Make a sauce with:
- 6 garlic cloves (finely minced)
- 4 tbsp. lemon juice
- 4 tbsp. mustard (any mustard)
- 3 tbsp. olive oil
- 1 tbsp. paprika
- Pinch of cayenne pepper
- 3 tbsp. honey
- 1 tsp. salt

Pour the sauce on the chicken, keep a little of it for later (about 4 tbsp.).

Marinate for at least 3 hours.

Grill the chicken over medium-high heat.

Serve on a platter and drizzle the rest of the sauce on top.

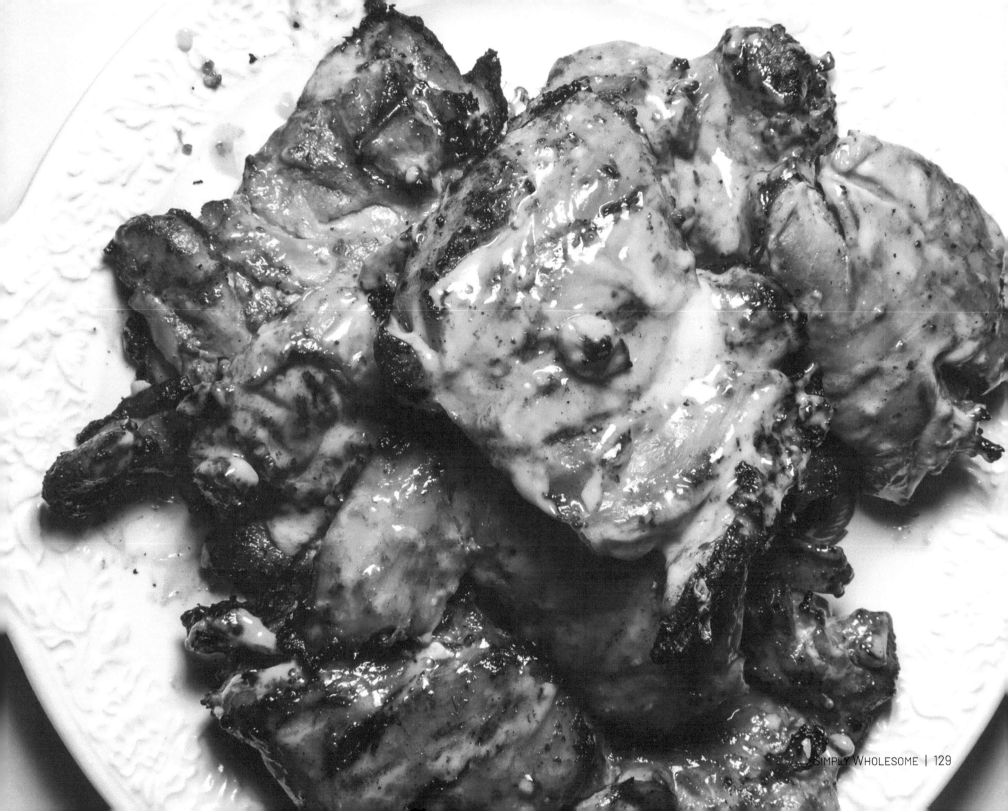

TILAPIA WITH TOMATO SAUCE

Ingredients

- 1 package frozen tilapia fillets
- 1/4 cup olive oil
- 1/2 cup tomato basil sauce
- Pinch of garlic powder, salt and pepper
- 1 onion, sliced into rings

Place the onion slices on the bottom of a 9 x 13 pan.
Place the tilapia on top.
Mix the sauce and pour on top of the fish.
Bake at 450 °F covered for 20 minutes, then uncovered for 5 minutes.

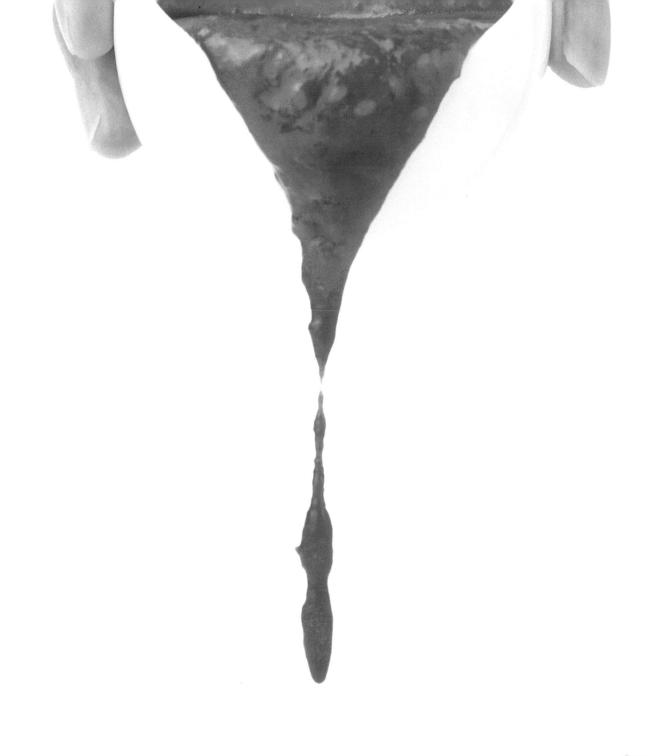

BEST GRILLED CHICKEN

This can be made on Pesach/Passover.

Ingredients

- 1 pack of chicken cutlets
- 12 frozen garlic cubes
- 12 frozen cilantro cubes
- 12 frozen basil cubes
- 1/8 cup Olive oil
- Pinch of salt

Add the other ingredients with the chicken cutlets in a zip lock bag and marinate for at least 2 hours, then grill.

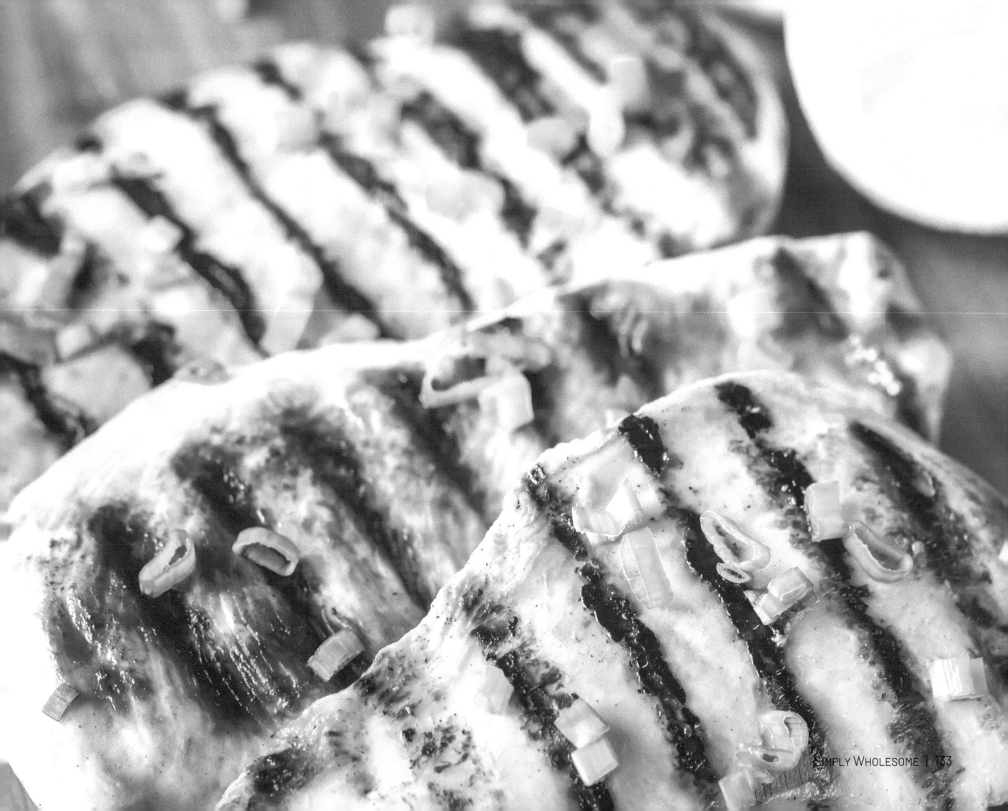

BROCCOLI CUTLETS

Ingredients

- 12 oz. broccoli florets—steamed
- 1 large egg + 1 egg white
- 1/2 cup chopped scallions
- 2/3 cup reduced-fat cheddar cheese
- 1/2 cup seasoned breadcrumbs/panko crumbs

Mix ingredients together and roll into small ovals.

Preheat oven to 400 °F.

Bake for 16 to 18 minutes.

Feel free to swap the broccoli with cauliflower.

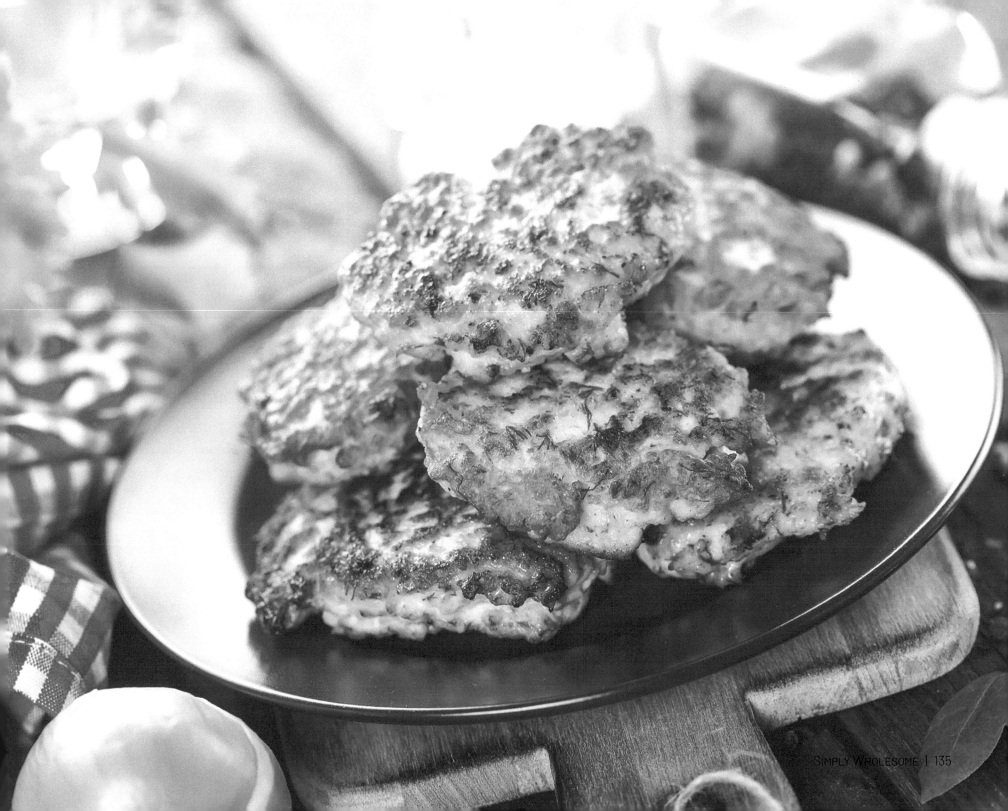

MELT-IN-YOUR-MOUTH GRILLED CHICKEN

Ingredients

- 1 package chicken cutlets, butterflied
- Light mayonnaise
- Smart Balance butter
- Trader Joe's Everything but The Bagel spice

Add 1 tbsp. of mayo around all the cutlets. Sprinkle the spice and smear each cutlet until coated.

Add the butter to the pan and wait until it melts.

Add all cutlets to the pan and cook until no longer pink and cooked through.

The butter makes these cutlets super soft and very juicy.

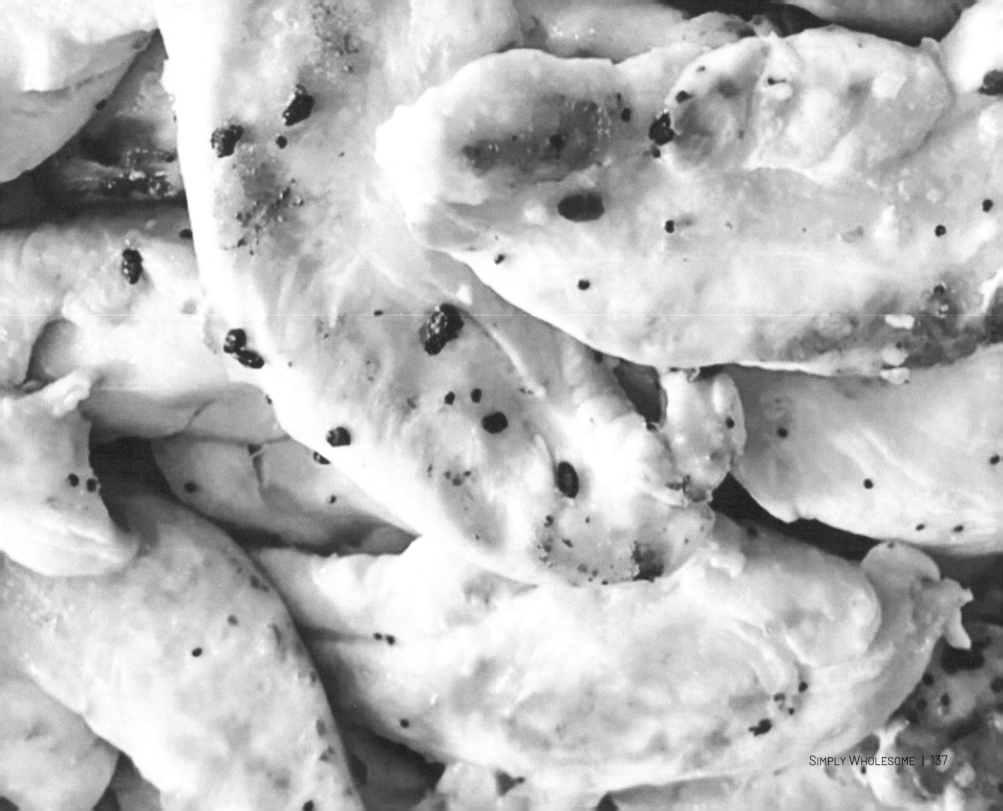

OVEN-ROASTED SALMON WITH LEMON PEPPER

- 1.3 lb. salmon with skin
- 1/2 lemon, juice only
- 2 tbsp. lemon pepper

Place the salmon skin side down in a roasting pan.
Squeeze over the juice from the lemon.
Spread out the lemon pepper evenly.
Now it's ready to go in the oven.
Bake for 20 minutes in the middle of the oven at 400 °F
Enjoy!

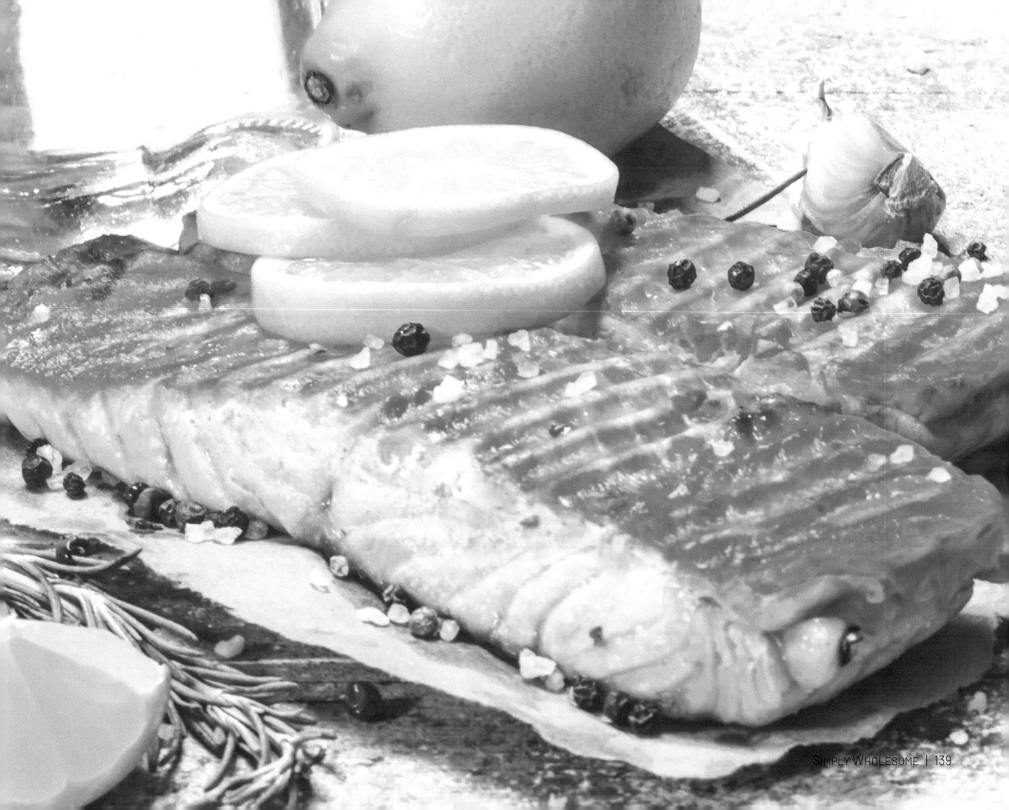

TURKEY MEATBALLS

Everyone in my family loves these, which is a miracle in and of itself!

Ingredients

- 1 lb. lean white ground turkey
- 1 egg
- Spices (onion powder, paprika, garlic, pepper, salt, and Montreal steak seasoning)
- 1/4 cup panko crumbs
- 1 24 oz. jar marinara sauce

Pour tomato sauce + water into pot. Shape ground turkey mixture (with the spices and egg) into balls. Cook 1 hour. Serve over brown rice, zoodles, etc.

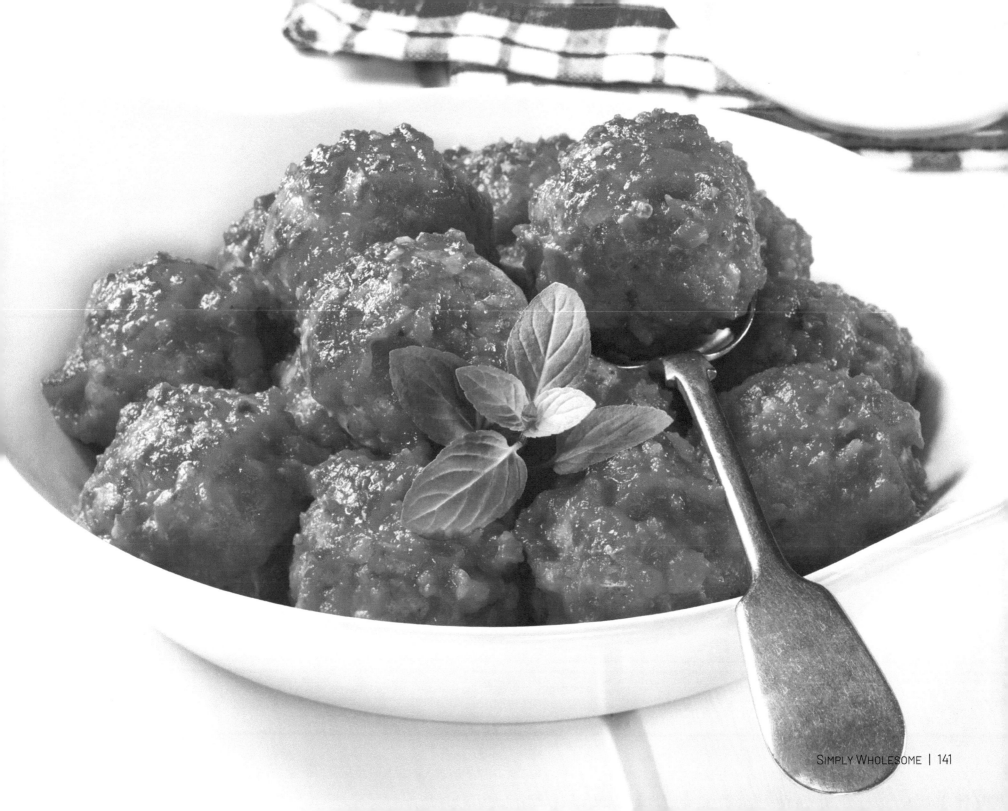

save room for dessert

- 6-ingredient protein brownies
- chocolate mousse
- chia seed pudding
- banana oatmeal cookies

- chocolate chip yogurt
- chocolate pudding
- strawberry cheesecake
- chickpeas cookies
- fruity ice pops

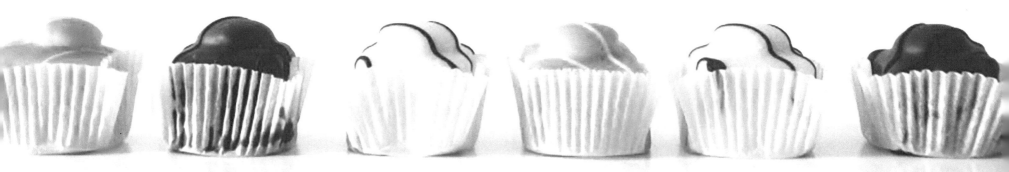

HELP YOURSELF TO

something sweet

6-INGREDIENT PROTEIN BROWNIES

Ingredients

- 1 banana
- 1/3 cup peanut butter
- 1/2 cup egg whites
- 3/4 cup unsweetened cocoa powder
- 2 scoops chocolate protein powder (I use whey)
- 3/4 cup unsweetened almond milk

Mash the banana and combine all ingredients together in a bowl. Mix until smooth.

Spray an 8 x 8 pan and bake at 350 °F for 20 minutes. (the top will be cracked). Let cool.

Drizzle with melted chocolate.

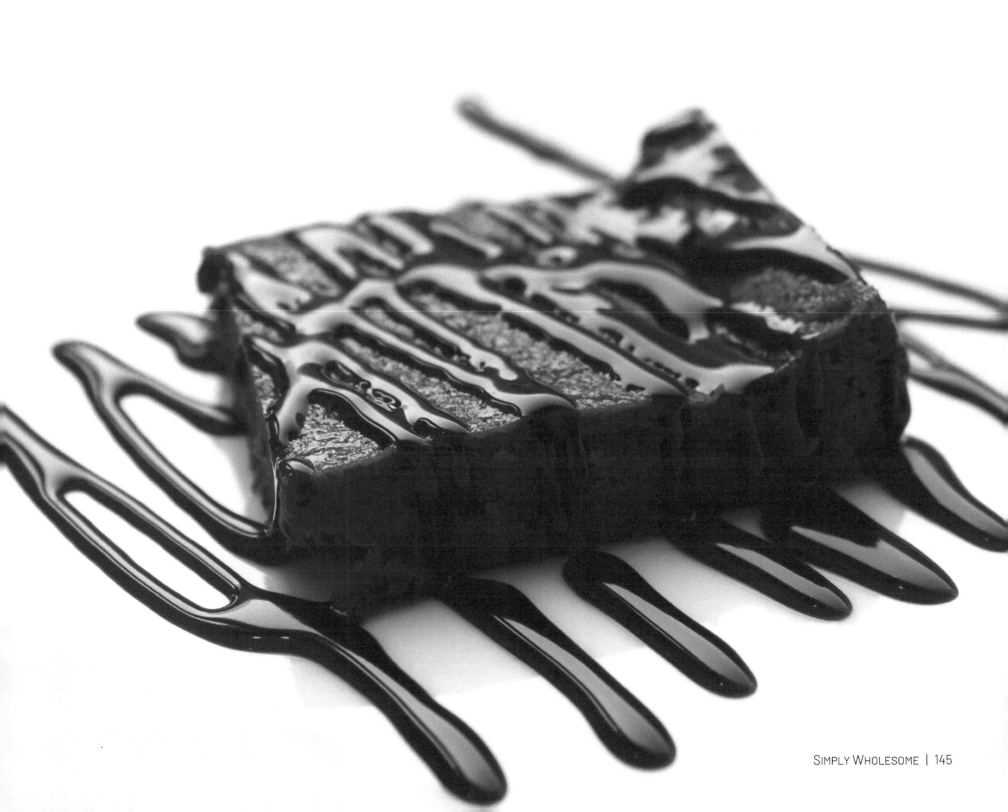

CHOCOLATE MOUSSE

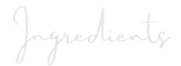

- 16 oz. unsweetened Greek yogurt
- 1/4 cup maple syrup
- 1/4 cup peanut (or almond) butter
- 1 bag (10 oz.) dark chocolate chips, melted
- 1/2 cup mini chocolate chips, (optional)

Blend yogurt, maple syrup, and peanut butter.

Melt chocolate chips in a double boiler (or microwave, mixing every 30 seconds).

Pour into blender and combine. Stir in the mini chocolate chips if desired.

Chill in the fridge for about 30 minutes. Top with chocolate shavings or whipped cream.

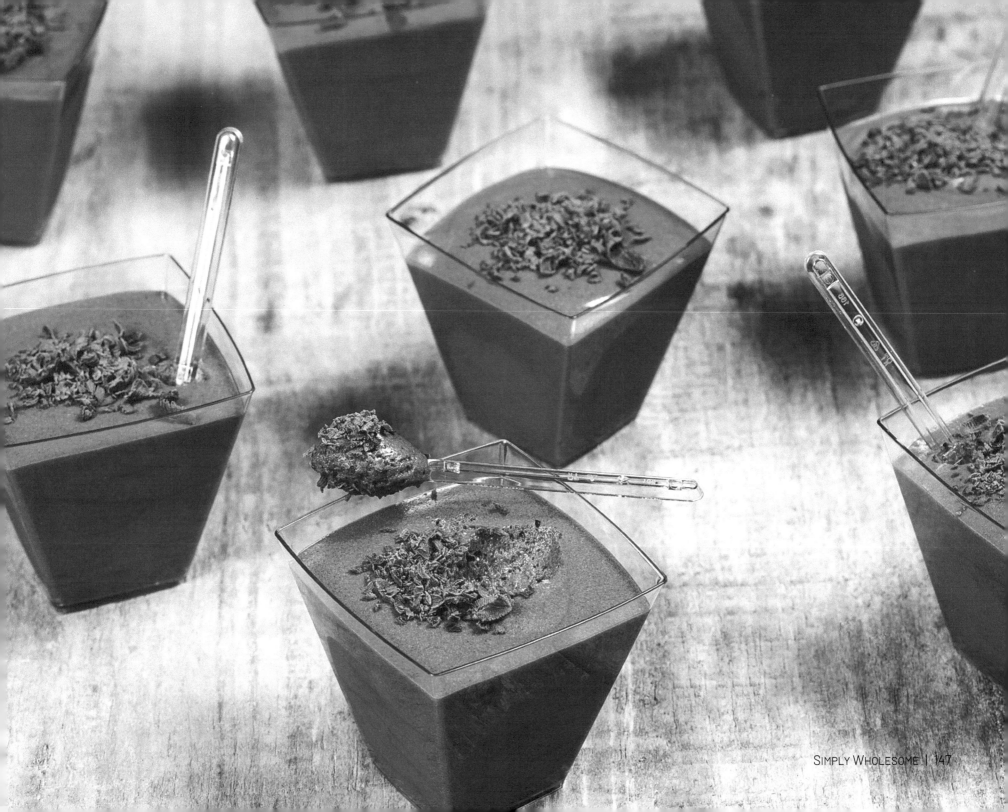

CHOCOLATE CHIA SEED PUDDING

Chia seeds are loaded with health benefits.
Packed with anti-oxidants, fiber, minerals, and Omega-3s, they are a great addition to your daily meals.

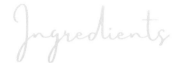

- 1 14 oz. unsweetened coconut milk
- 1/3 cup chia seeds
- 1/4 cup maple syrup
- 3 tbsp. unsweetened cocoa powder
- 1 tsp. vanilla extract
- 1/4 cup coconut flakes
- raspberries or blueberries, for topping

In a bowl combine the ingredients, except berries. Whisk together and chill for 3 hours.
Serve into bowls and top with berries.

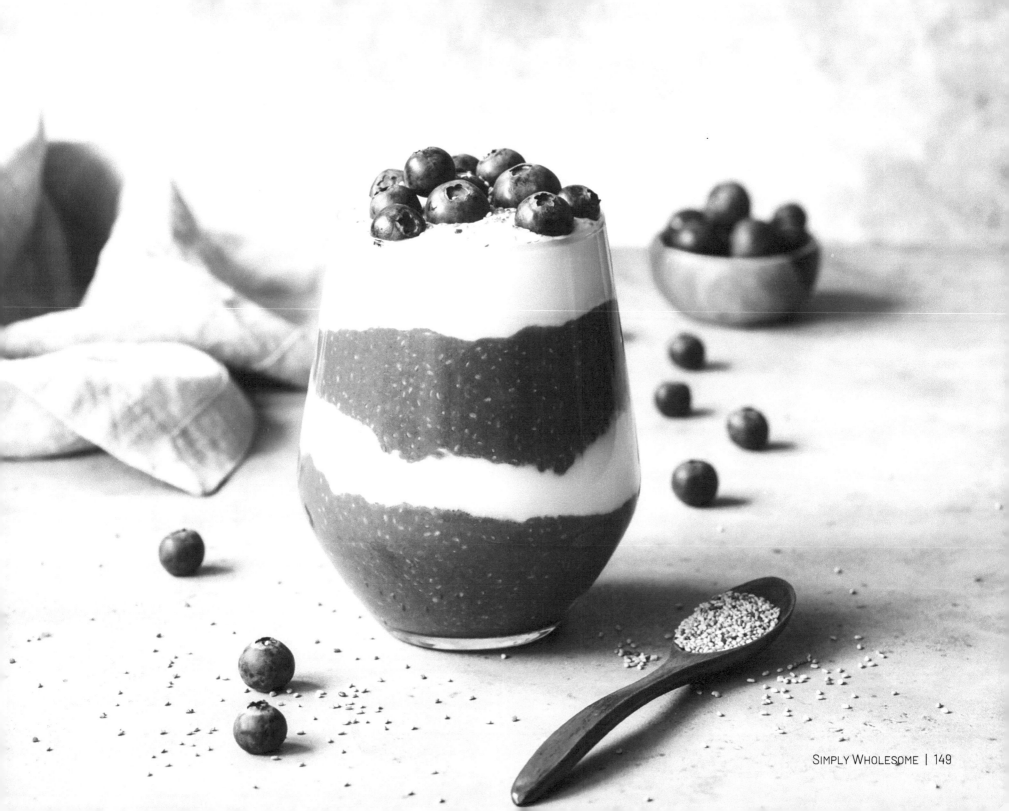

3-INGREDIENT BANANA OATMEAL COOKIES

Ingredients

- 2 medium ripe bananas, mashed
- 1 cup of uncooked quick oats
- 1/4 cup crushed walnuts

Preheat oven to 350 °F. Combine the mashed bananas and oats in a bowl. Fold in the walnuts.
Place a tablespoon of each on the cookie sheet.
Bake 15 minutes. Makes 16 cookies.

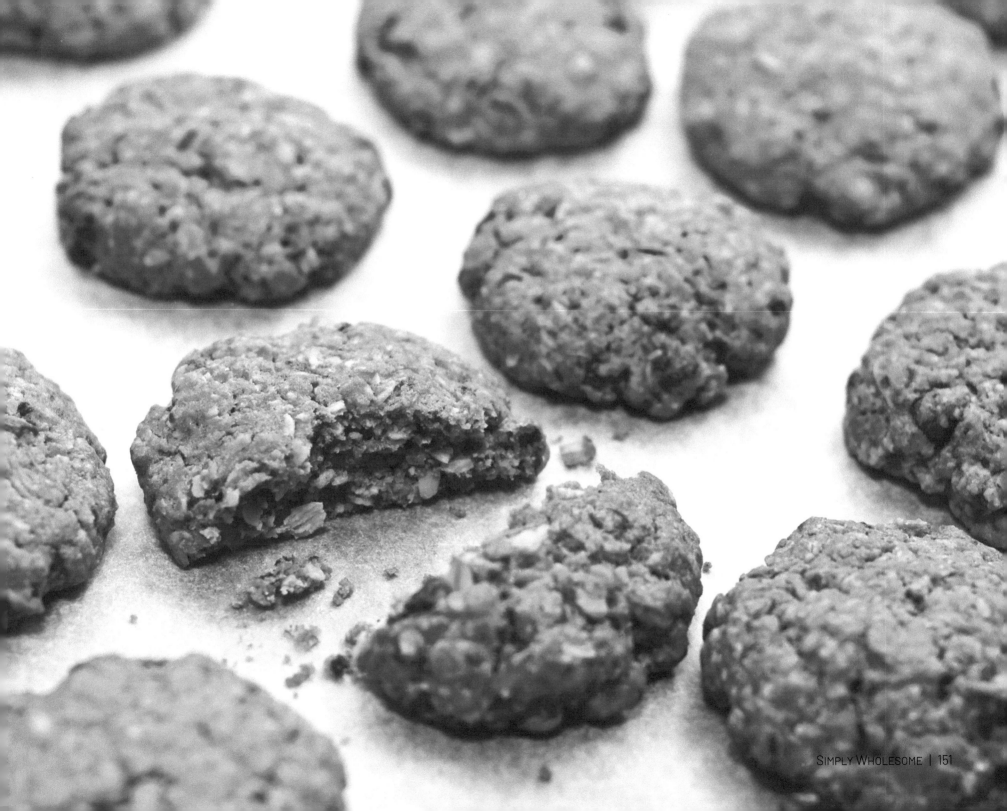

CHOCOLATE CHIP GREEK YOGURT

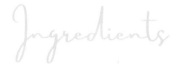

Ingredients

- 6 oz. greek yogurt
- 1 tbsp. peanut or other nut butter
- 1/2 tsp. vanilla extract
- 1/4 tsp. almond extract
- 1–2 tsp. chocolate chips

In a small/medium bowl, whisk together all of the ingredients until smooth.

Top with chocolate chips or chocolate shavings, if desired.

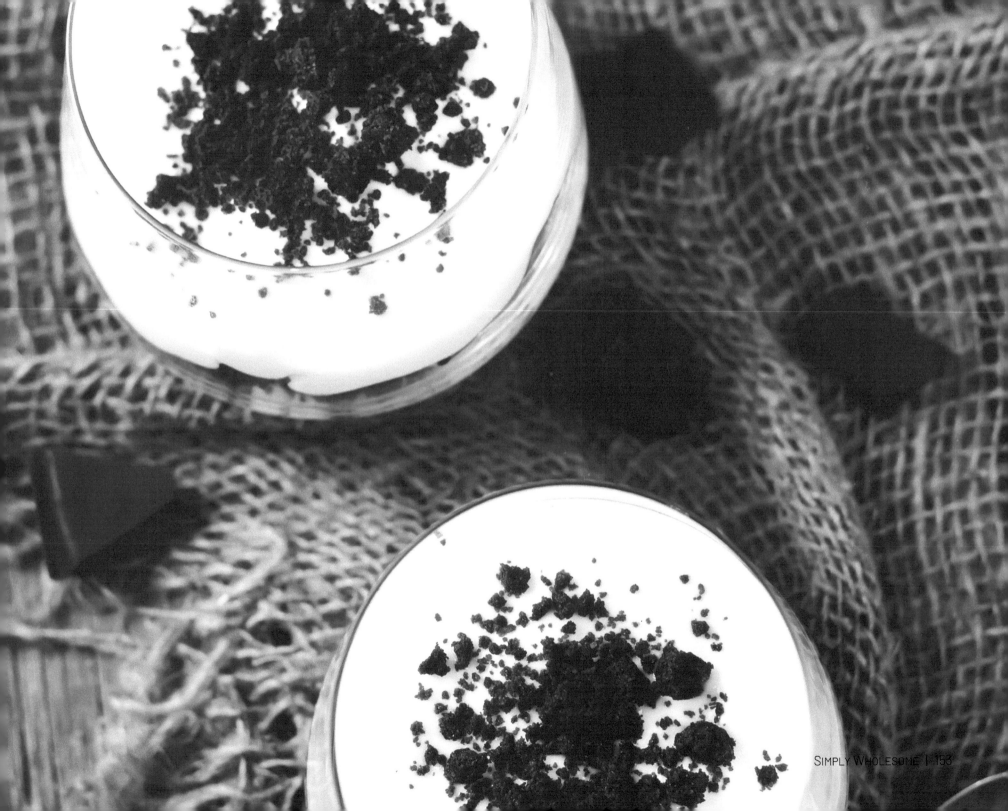

CHOCOLATE PUDDING

This pudding is so good. I actually couldn't believe it at first. The avocado makes it thick, but you don't taste it.

Ingredients

- 1 cup unsweetened almond milk
- 1/4–1/2 avocado (for thickness)
- 2 tbsp. unsweetened cocoa powder
- 1 tbsp. stevia or truvia
- 2 squares of any sugar-free chocolate (I used ChocoPerfection from Amazon)
- Ice

Blend all ingredients **except** the chocolate squares. Add that afterwards and only blend for 30 seconds. You should still see bits of chocolate. Refrigerate.

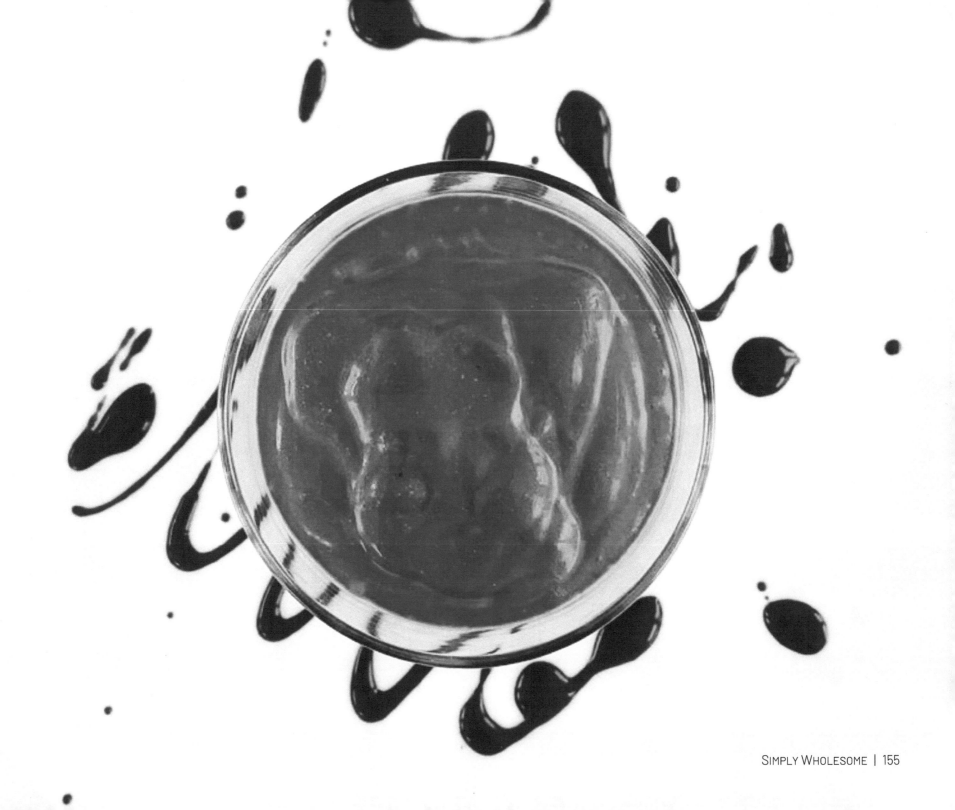

STRAWBERRY CHEESECAKE

Perfect for Shavous or any other time!

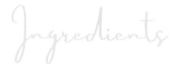

Ingredients

- Cooking spray
- 1/2 cup crushed pecans
- 1 tbsp. honey
- 8 oz. reduced-fat cream cheese
- 1/4 cup truvia/stevia
- 6 oz. vanilla Greek yogurt
- 2 large egg whites
- 2 tbsp. lemon juice
- 1/2 tsp. vanilla extract
- 1 tbsp. all-purpose flour
- 1/4 cup low-sugar strawberry jam

Preheat oven to 350 °F. Coat a non-stick square baking pan with non-stick spray.

Mix together crushed pecans and honey with a fork until evenly moistened. Press evenly into bottom of prepared pan.

Gently beat cream cheese, sugar, and vanilla using electric mixer.

Gradually beat in yogurt, egg whites, lemon juice, and flour. Do not over beat. Pour over pecan crust.

Stir jam until smooth. Drop small spoonfuls over surface of cheesecake filling.

Using a knife, swirl gently through filling to create a marble effect.

Bake for 50–55 minutes, uncovered.

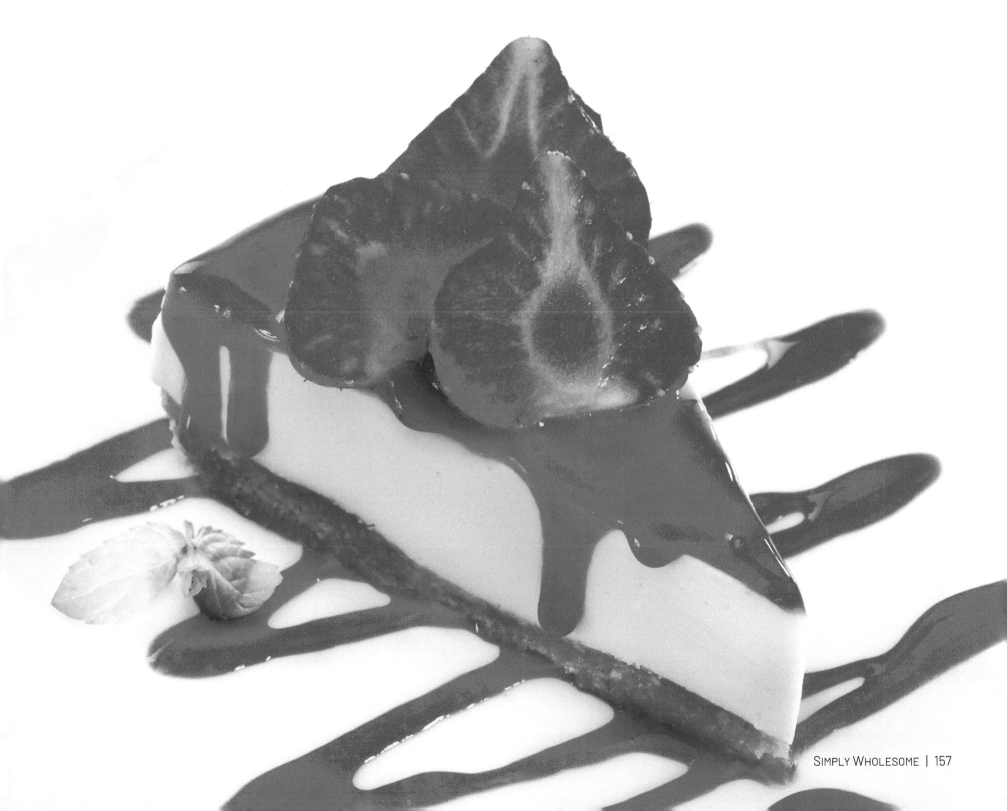

CHOCOLATE CHICKPEA COOKIES

You do not taste the chickpeas in these at all. Hands down, best cookies—preferably straight out of the oven!

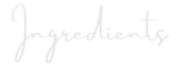

- 1 can chickpeas, drained
- 3 tbsp. flour, I used whole wheat
- 4 tbsp. sugar, I used truvia
- 2 tbsp. coconut oil
- 2 tsp. vanilla
- 1/4 tsp. baking soda and powder
- 1/2 tsp. salt
- 1/3 cup chocolate chips (optional)

Preheat oven to 350 °F.

Place chickpeas in food processor and blend for 5 minutes.

Blend rest of ingredients for 2 minutes.

Add in chocolate chips.

Place small-sized droppings onto baking sheet.

Bake for 15–18 minutes.

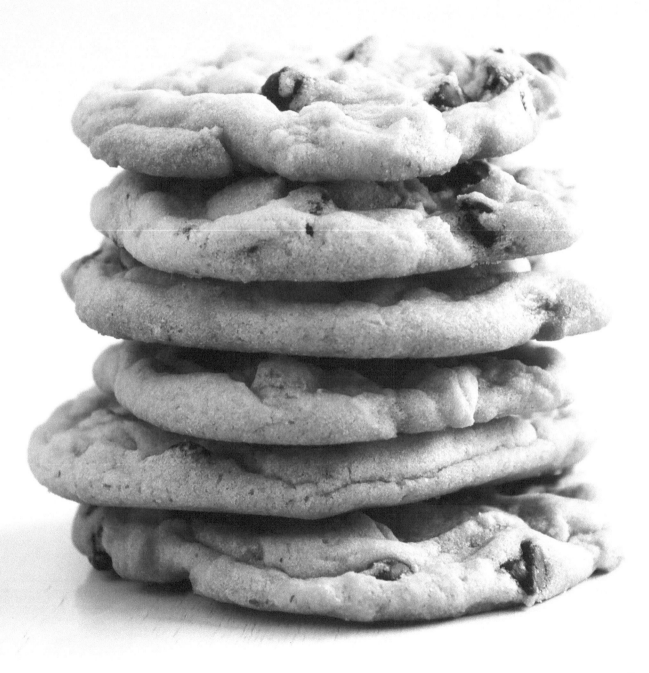

FRUITY ICE POPS

Perfect for that hot humid afternoon in the summer, when you just want to cool off. These ice pops do just that.

Ingredients

- 6 strawberries
- 3 kiwis
- 1 cup unsweetened almond milk

Blend all ingredients. Pour into ice pop molds and freeze.

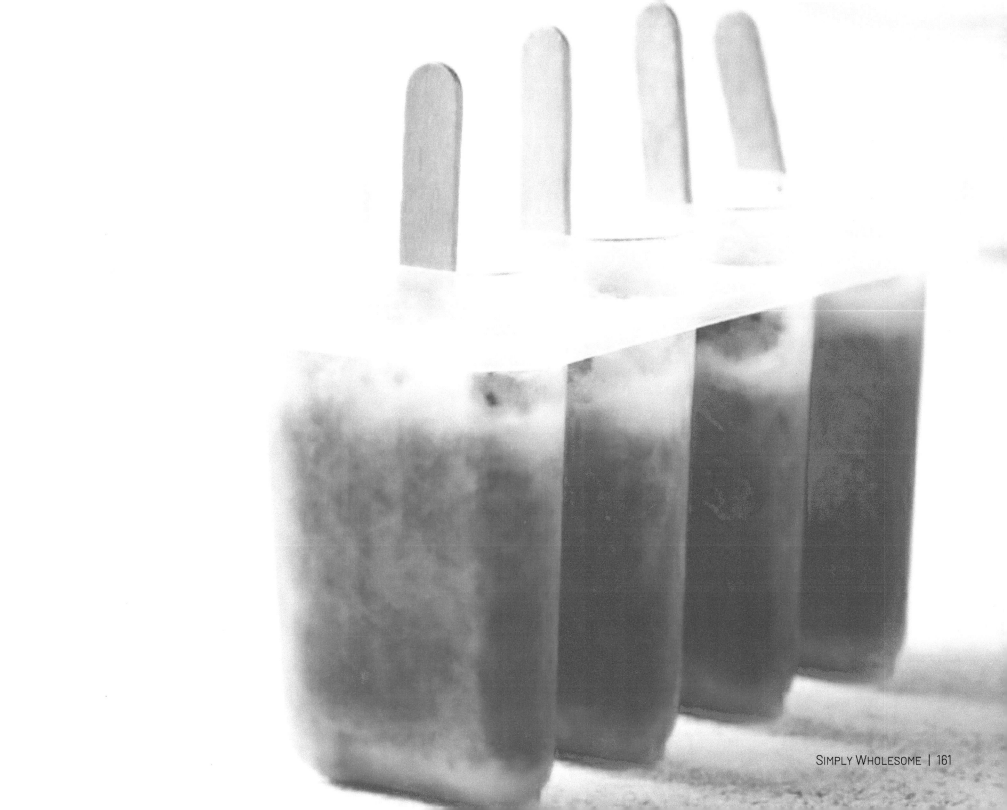

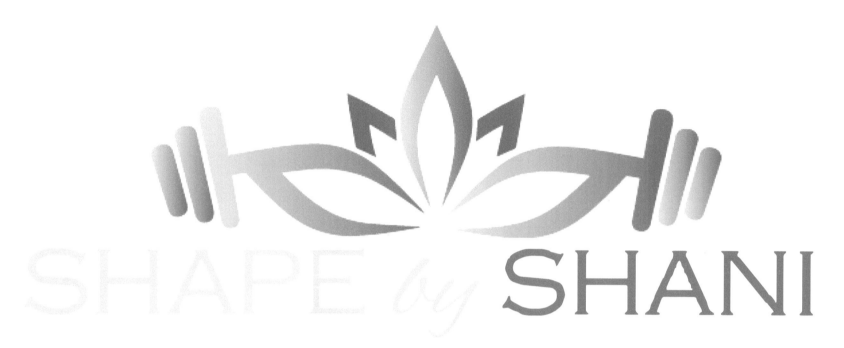

SHAPE by SHANI

Not Just Fitness...Wellness

SCAN ME

CPSIA information can be obtained
at www.ICGtesting.com
Printed in the USA
LVHW020956211222
735678LV00015B/519